W9-CCE-668

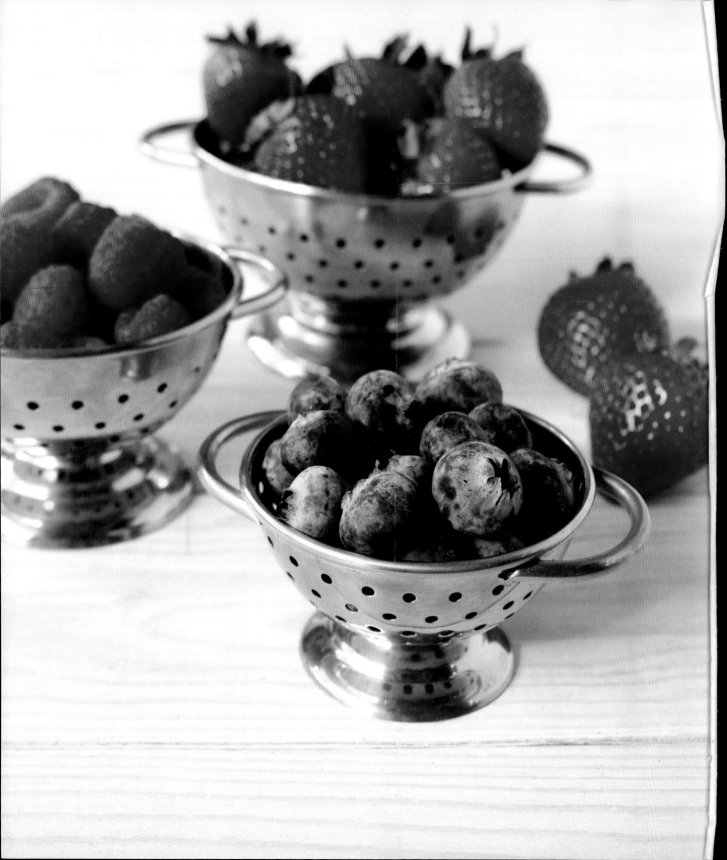

Glow

Introduction

• • •

YOUR CONCEALER CALLED

IT WANTS A DAY OFF

Oh, to think of the countless hours I spent mediating the daily battle between my concealer and my blemishes!

The miles I walked, pacing the drugstore beauty aisle in search of the Holy Grail that would make everything right. The tears I cried over my "troubled" skin—surely enough to fill a bathtub so I could bathe in my own sorrow.

Okay, yes, so I'm being a little dramatic. But if you've ever been desperate for smooth, clear, glowing skin, then you feel my pain.

Unfortunately, most of us look for the solution to our skincare woes in all the wrong places. We look to lotions and potions and pills. People to scrub and peel and pop. All drama aside, I shudder to think about the crazy things I used to put on my face—from countless prescriptions to sketchy skin peels purchased off the Internet. At one point, I was applying rubbing alcohol morning and night in an attempt to kill every last acne-causing bacteria. What did these do for me? Only further inflame my already irritated skin and add to my body burden. Because not only were these products filled with unhealthy chemicals, they were stripping my skin of its natural protective oils rather than helping to soothe and repair the skin. Most importantly, they didn't address the root cause of the problem, but were merely trying to cover it up.

Truly healthy skin is not something we can find in a bottle or jar. It's an inside job. It begins with health.

Looking back, it makes complete sense that I got acne when I did, though at the time I was so ridiculously gosh darn confused. I had perfect skin all through my teens, and wasn't that the time I was supposed to be breaking out? Hadn't I already graduated from the stage of life when acne was a concern? I was still using the same products that kept my skin smooth and clear as a teenager—why weren't they working? The problem wasn't that puberty struck me later in life or that my trusty skincare routine had suddenly started to fail. It was that everything happening behind the scenes in my body had changed, and not for the better: My diet included a lot of processed "health" foods that were lacking in skin-supporting nutrients and causing chronic inflammation, my digestive system was thrown into a state of chaos after multiple rounds of antibiotics and my hormones were totally out of whack thanks to sky-high stress levels and a stressed-out liver. Each of these takes its toll on the skin. And combined with my harsh "anti-acne" skincare routine, it was a recipe for disaster.

After learning about my "body burden," I became impassioned to adopt a healthier, natural lifestyle, including skincare. It all started with a little conversation with my sister.

SISTER: "Have you heard about these things called parabens? Apparently they're pretty bad for you. I looked and they're in a lot of my lotions and shampoos and stuff."

ME: "I don't believe you."

BUT I CHECKED AND SHE WAS RIGHT: These chemicals had been found to interfere with specific hormones (you know, the chemical messengers that control our major bodily functions) and they were in each and every one of my products, too. After that, I became feverish to learn more about the harmful chemicals that were such an intimate part of my life yet complete strangers. What I learned was shocking and inspired me to start my website, Body Unburdened, which has since helped hundreds of thousands of readers learn about their exposure to these chemicals and simple solutions for a healthier lifestyle.

ONE FACT THAT REALLY BLEW ME AWAY: On the average day, the average woman comes into contact with over 150 chemicals via her skincare and beauty products. Yes, daily! Like parabens, some of these chemicals are known endocrine-disruptors (i.e., they mess with your hormones) or have been linked to an increased risk of cancer. Even more concerning, most of these chemicals have not been studied for safety due to loopholes in chemical safety laws.

So, instilled with this knowledge, I threw away all of my old chemical-filled products and replaced them with new nontoxic alternatives. And . . . I didn't see any difference in my skin. This is because I was still completely ignoring my diet and everything else happening inside my body. Fortunately, not long after detoxing my skincare routine I had a lightbulb moment: I realized this was just one small aspect of my health.

My skin finally started to improve when I focused on nourishing it from the inside out.

It's time to put down the concealer and pick up the fork.

What if you could fight the signs of aging, soothe and smooth your skin by making simple adjustments to your diet? Are you already licking your lips?

Well, it's time we learn that beauty is not only skin deep—the skin is a mirror that reflects internal imbalances. It's as simple and as complicated as that: simple because, once we know which imbalances in particular are triggering our skin issues, we can work to remedy them; complicated because that doesn't happen at the snap of a finger and can sometimes take quite a bit of detective work to uncover. But the work required to remedy these imbalances will be so worth it, and not just for beauty's sake. Common skin issues are often caused by a lack of proper nutrition, blood sugar dysregulation, inflammation, poor digestion and impaired gut health and hormonal imbalances, each of which has significant implications beyond skin health. And so, skin issues can be seen as a good thing (I bet you've never thought of your zits or eczema in that way before!) since they are often a symptom that is cluing you in to an internal imbalance that needs to be corrected. They're telling you, "Hey, something is wrong here!"

So if you've had enough of all of the lotions and potions, I'm here to tell you that these are not the best way to get clear, healthy, glowing skin anyway. A healthy diet is the best and surest way to the skin of your dreams. And a simple, natural approach to topical skincare is the cherry on top.

We all deserve to love the skin we're in.

And it's not about vanity or being the prettiest at the party. It's about confidence and being comfortable in your own body. It's about literally putting your best face forward to take on the world.

My hope in writing this book is for you to feel empowered to take control of your health and your skin, which are very intimately connected. Depending on where you are in your personal health journey, it may require a bit of effort. But the greatest investment you will ever make is in your health. So, with every bit of effort you expend, know that you are investing in a healthier body, and that this investment will pay off in dividends—one such reward being naturally gorgeous, glowing skin from within.

BEFORE WE GET STARTED . . .

LET'S LEVEL WITH EACH OTHER

Let's talk about what you will and will not get out of this book.

YOU'LL GET:

- An in-depth knowledge of how the skin works. This will include a little anatomy lesson, but trust me: It's totally fascinating. Plus, knowing exactly how this organ works is vital to understanding where things go wrong and how to set them right again.

- To know the common culprits behind most skin issues plus how to remedy them. Bonus: These are the same bad boys behind most chronic health ailments and diseases, so this knowledge will benefit your body far beyond skin health.

- A deep understanding of the best-kept secret for gorgeous, glowing skin: proper nutrition. You'll learn how to leverage nutrition and nourish your body to benefit the skin, but in doing so will get a comprehensive knowledge of proper nutrition basics.

- A lesson in how to appropriately care for your skin from the outside. We'll discuss the unhealthy ingredients found in most conventional skincare products, my favorite topic—body burden—and why a natural approach to skincare is best. And of course, we'll talk about safer skincare options, including those you can make yourself.

- Twenty yummy skin-loving superfood recipes plus twenty all-natural do-it-yourself skincare recipes. The food recipes are meant to help as you work to transform your diet to one that nourishes your body and fosters glowing skin from within. They're all quite simple and include nutrients that the skin adores. And if you know me at all, you know I love a good skincare DIY! Again, these are all rather simple (some shockingly so) and use a number of the same ingredients so you can create a variety of homemade skincare products without breaking the bank.

YOU WON'T GET:

- A magic bullet, one-stop-shop "cure" for skin issues and ailments. Unfortunately, that just doesn't exist! Our individual bodies vary so greatly, and what causes skin issues (even the same skin issues) varies from person to person. The good news? A healthy diet can remedy the causes of most common skin issues. I'll show you how.

HOW YOU CAN MAKE THE MOST OF THIS BOOK

YOUR BODY IS DIFFERENT FROM MY BODY IS DIFFERENT FROM HER BODY IS DIFFERENT FROM HIS

Keep in mind: We're all unique individuals!

This is true for our biology as well as our beliefs.

As we'll discuss, some very nutritious foods, such as eggs or tomatoes, don't sit very well with some individuals who have an allergy or intolerance. Similarly, some people will choose to avoid certain foods for religious or ethical reasons, or simply because they don't like them!

For these reasons, all the nutritional information contained in this book is meant to provide you with a foundational knowledge of how to nourish your body for glowing skin from within. You are free to take the information and make it work for your unique life and skin needs.

It's important to take a long and hard look at your current diet and lifestyle to understand how different foods may be affecting your body and skin.

To make the most of this book, it's important to be in tune with your body and listen closely for the messages it's sending you. The best way to do this is with a food journal. This super simple tool helps you recognize the connection between certain foods and the way you look and feel.

I encourage you to:

1. Keep a food journal for three days with your current diet. Yes, I'm suggesting that you go on eating and drinking whatever it is you typically eat and drink for three more days, even if it's really, really bad! This is important for two reasons: It can help you recognize (1) "Hmm, I don't eat nearly as well as I thought I did," which is key to making positive changes, and (2) "Oh goodness, that food really makes me look and feel icky," which is key to avoiding relapse.

2. As you begin working to nourish your skin from the inside by applying what you learn in this book, keep a new food journal for another three days. This will help you recognize the positive impact your new diet is having on your skin and overall wellness. Wait one to two weeks after you start the new diet to begin this second journal since you may experience an adjustment period during this time (weaning yourself off sugar and introducing healthy probiotics, for example, can cause slight detox or healing reactions for some individuals; this is a hurdle that must be jumped but not an indication of how this new dietary approach will make you look and feel in the long run).

3. Compare your food journals and make note of your progress. Be sure to give yourself a pat on the back and blow a kiss at yourself in the mirror! Feel empowered to have control over your skin and health and proud for making this tremendous investment in your well-being.

In a notebook or on a blank piece of paper, create your three-day food journal. Include everything you eat and drink, including water. Don't skip a thing! No one else is looking at this and judging you, so be completely honest—it's important for you to get an accurate picture of what exactly is going into your body on a daily basis, so you can make positive, effective changes. Be sure to note how you feel and at what time of day. This includes both physical feelings—stomachache, nausea, gas, headache—as well as energy levels and mood—tired, sad, jittery, anxious. Feeling lethargic in the afternoon or having a stomachache right after breakfast are important clues into how your diet is affecting your body, including your skin!

PARTICULAR THINGS TO LOOK OUT FOR:

- The amount and variety of real foods
- The amount and quality of each macronutrient
- The amount of water and diuretic beverages
- The amount of omega-6 and omega-3 essential fatty acids
- Correlations between certain foods and digestive distress, aches and pains, sleep patterns, changes in the skin or any other physical change

If you're wondering what some of these terms mean, don't worry—we'll be going over them all in just a bit!

The chart on the next page shows a sample of one day's food journal entry.

TIME	I ATE	I DRANK (OZ)	I FEEL	MY SKIN IS
8 A.M.	Berry Satisfying Chia Pudding Parfait (page 99)	4 oz (120 ml) water	Energized	Broken out around my mouth and chin
10 A.M.	-----	8 oz (240 ml) coffee with coconut milk	A little bloated	-----
11 A.M.	Handful of walnuts	8 oz (240 ml) water	-----	-----
1 P.M.	Sweet and Savory Butternut Squash Chili (page 88)	2 oz (60 ml) water	-----	-----
3 P.M.	2 oz (60 g) dark chocolate	8 oz (240 ml) water	Tired	Really oily
7 P.M.	Baked "Spaghetti" Pie (page 92)	-----	-----	-----
8 P.M.	Tropical Turmeric Ice Pops (page 112)	8 oz (240 ml) water	-----	-----

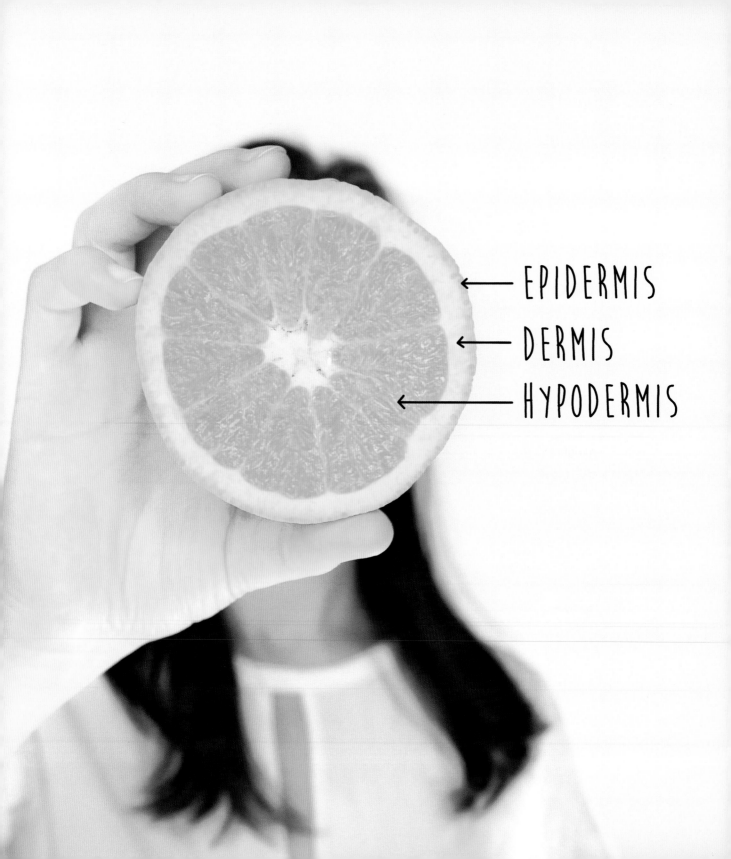

EPIDERMIS

DERMIS

HYPODERMIS

Understanding the Skin

• • •

YOUR BODY'S LARGEST ORGAN 101

PLEASE ALLOW ME TO INTRODUCE YOU

The skin is a truly amazing organ that plays a number of important roles in the body.

Pump the brakes. My skin is an organ?

Yep! The skin is actually your body's largest organ. And in my personal opinion, one of the most fascinating. Knowing how it works is key to understanding where things go wrong and how we can make them right again.

The skin does a lot more than simply keep all of our insides wrapped up (though that in itself is very important). It controls the body's core temperature and is the body's first line of defense from outside intruders, such as bacteria and allergens, making it a key player in the body's immune system. The skin is also your body's main source of vitamin D, an absolutely critical vitamin to health and vitality—the skin synthesizes vitamin D when exposed to the sun's ultraviolet (UV) rays.

SOME FUN FACTS ABOUT THE SKIN

- The average adult has about 20 square feet (1.9 m²) of skin weighing 10 pounds (4.5 kg).
- Our skin sheds 30,000 to 40,000 dead skin cells every minute (whoa).

The anatomy of the skin is all about layers.

The skin has three main layers: the epidermis, the dermis and the hypodermis (or subcutaneous fat layer). It helps to think of the skin and its layers as an orange: The epidermis is the very thin, bright orange part of the peel; the dermis is the thicker, white part of the peel that's visible when you cut the orange; and the hypodermis is the pulp of the fruit.

THE EPIDERMIS has many of its own layers and contains four principal types of cells, though it's less than 1 millimeter thick. About 90 percent of the epidermis is composed of keratinocytes, which make the protein keratin and are rapidly dividing. Keratin is a very strong protein that acts as a barrier and protects the skin from microbes, heat and abrasions. Another roughly 8 percent of epidermal cells are melanocytes, the cells that produce melanin. Melanin gives the skin its pigment and absorbs UV light from the sun. The epidermis also contains tactile cells, which detect the sensation of touch, and Langerhans cells, which are an important part of the body's immune system and launch immune responses against invading microbes.

Unlike most other organs, the skin is constantly renewing itself.

As the keratinocytes divide and multiply, they crowd out the older cells. These older cells are pushed up and eventually shed as dead skin cells. This is *great news* for anyone struggling with a skin issue since it means that the skin you currently have will be gone in about a month's time, replaced by totally new cells.

THE DERMIS is mainly composed of collagen and elastin, proteins that give the skin strength and structure. Collagen makes up about 70 percent of the dermis, while elastin holds the collagen in place and keeps the skin flexible. The dermis is also home to nerve receptors, blood vessels, sweat and oil glands and hair follicles—an absolute ton of them! The average square inch of skin contains more than 1,000 nerve receptors, 20 blood vessels, 650 sweat glands and 65 hair follicles (I told you it was fascinating).

THE HYPODERMIS is the fatty layer that covers the muscles, insulates the body and provides cushioning. It contains nerve endings and large blood vessels that supply the upper layers of the skin.

Where do pores come into this picture?

We can't look at our skin without seeing pores, those little tiny holes that are a source of unending frustration for so many of us. Well, when you see a pore, you're actually looking at a hair shaft.

A hair is nothing more than a thread of dead skin cells fused together (which is why when you work on creating beautiful skin from the inside, fabulous hair is likely to be a welcomed side effect). The root penetrates into the dermis and is surrounded by a hair follicle that is made of epidermal cells. Sebaceous (oil) glands are connected to the hair follicles and also housed in the dermis. They secrete sebum, the skin's natural oil, into the hair follicle. Sebum has a purpose other than creating a lucrative market for blotting papers and mattifying powders—it is meant to keep hair and skin moisturized, prevent water from evaporating from the skin and to inhibit the growth of certain bacteria. Problems occur, however, when the hair shaft becomes clogged with dead skin cells. This causes the sebum to get backed up in the pore and the sebaceous gland to inflame. This creates what we lovingly call a zit.

Pore size is unfortunately mostly determined by genetics (thanks a lot, Mom and Dad). However, you can take measures to prevent pores from sagging and appearing larger, as typically happens with age and free radical damage. Topical products with astringent properties can help pores temporarily appear smaller, but cannot permanently reduce pore size.

Sitting atop the skin is a fascinating little world in and of itself.

The skin's sebum creates a protective barrier called the acid mantle on the surface of the skin. The acid mantle has a distinct, slightly acidic pH that must be maintained. Let's go back to middle school science class for a moment: The pH scale is used to identify the acidity or alkalinity of a liquid and runs from 0 to 14, with 0 being acidic, 7 being neutral and 14 being alkaline. The pH of the skin's acid mantle is around 5.5. This is the skin's happy place. This is the pH at which all is calm and peaceful. If the acid mantle is disrupted, bad bacteria are allowed to thrive and the skin's shedding process may be disrupted. This is especially important to keep in mind when considering topical skincare products, as many have a more alkaline pH and so can irritate the skin by shifting the pH of the acid mantle away from its happy place.

Within the acid mantle is the skin's own microbiome. This is really just a fancy name to represent all of the bacteria living on our skin. Now don't get the heebie-jeebies, but it's estimated that there are over 1,000 different species of bacteria living on the skin! It's very important to know that not all of these bacteria are bad. In fact, few are and others are even believed to benefit the skin.

COMMON SKIN ISSUES DEFINED

YOU KNOW WHAT THEY SAY: KNOW YOUR ENEMY

Your skin is not your enemy! What's happening to it is.

Let's take a look at some common skincare issues, so we can better understand how to support our skin with nutrition and natural skincare.

ACNE

We know what pimples are: OBNOXIOUS! But what are they really? When it comes down to it, a zit is nothing more than a sticky mess of dead skin cells and/or dirt and the skin's natural oil trapped within a pore. The famous *Propionibacterium acnes* (*P. acnes*) bacteria then feast on this sticky mess. It's important to know that everyone has the P. acnes bacteria living on their skin, even those individuals with nearly flawless, movie-star skin. It's when a pore becomes clogged that *P. acnes* starts to become a problem—the bacteria quickly multiply and break down the sebum into irritating fatty acids. This causes the sebaceous gland to inflame, resulting in redness, swelling and pain.

Although the finger is often pointed at *P. acnes* as the cause of acne, there's *a lot* more to it. The large majority of acne sufferers are diligently washing their face and applying topical bacteria-fighting products, but they continue to suffer from breakouts because the bacteria is often not the primary cause. As you will soon learn, there is a lot going on within their bodies that is perpetuating their skin troubles.

AGING

Aging is a natural process and not one I am trying to stop. In fact, one of my favorite quotes is: "Do not regret growing older; it is a privilege denied to many." Life truly is a privilege and should be celebrated, not condemned. None of this "Oh, it's my 20th 20th birthday" garbage! You're 40 and should be darn proud of that! That being said, I'd like to "age gracefully" and certainly not before my time, and I'm sure you agree.

Most skin aging happens in the dermis. You'll recall that this is where collagen and elastin are housed, and that these two proteins keep skin flexible and elastic. Aging is characterized by the reduced ability of cells to repair or replace damaged cells. As collagen and elastin stiffen, break and decrease in number due to reduced cellular division and repair, wrinkles and furrows form. This is why the expression lines around our mouth and eyes and on our forehead eventually become ever-present wrinkles—the skin loses its resilience and ability to bounce back into place.

Unless you never move your face (and I don't think that would be a very fun way to go through life!), wrinkles are inevitable. But there are a number of factors that accelerate skin aging, which we can take precautions to reduce. We can even boost the repair and production of collagen and elastin.

ECZEMA

This inflammatory condition produces dry, itchy patches of skin. Although it most often appears on the arms and legs, eczema can affect any part of the skin. Often, bouts of eczema flare and wane, and seem to be connected to allergies, though no cause of eczema has been medically defined.

Chicken skin or *keratosis pilaris* is a specific type of eczema that affects approximately 50 percent of adults. It appears most often on the back of the arms as rough, pink bumps.

ROSACEA

There's a big difference between a shy blush and this inflammatory skin condition. Rosacea causes the skin to flush and turn red for extended periods of time and can be very uncomfortable. Skin sensitivity, broken blood vessels and small pimples may accompany the flushing. Most individuals begin experiencing rosacea in their late teens or twenties, with an increase in severity during their thirties and forties. There is no known medically defined cause of rosacea, but spicy foods, alcohol, exercise and heat seem to trigger flares.

SUN DAMAGE

The sun's UV rays create free radicals in the skin that cause inflammation and damage the structural proteins of the skin, leading to "photoaging"—accelerated aging as a result of sun exposure. Free radicals also damage DNA, which can lead to cancer. To protect itself from these damaging effects, the skin increases its production of melanin in response to sunlight. This is why the skin turns tan. Sometimes, there is an uneven increase in melanin production, resulting in "sun spots."

This is a tricky subject, since the body requires the skin to be exposed to sunlight to synthesize the critically important vitamin D. Luckily, there are ways to practice safe sun exposure so you can produce adequate vitamin D while also protecting the skin from UV damage.

DRY SKIN

Dry skin can be caused by a lack of moisture or a lack of hydration. They kind of sound like the same thing, right? But skin moisture has to do with oil, whereas hydration has to do with water. Skin that lacks moisture tends to be rough or flaky, whereas dehydrated skin looks dull and feels tight.

The amount of water we drink most greatly influences skin hydration, whereas dietary fats influence moisture, but skincare also plays a key role—the wrong products will dehydrate and strip the skin of its natural oils that keep water locked in the skin. The skin also produces less sebum as we age, which can cause dryness.

OILY SKIN

Although oil is a natural and necessary part of the skin, its production can sometimes get kicked into overdrive. There are a number of different reasons that this may happen. As we will learn, specific hormones and specific foods that increase the production of these hormones can stimulate oil production. It is also common for the skin to produce more oil in response to harsh, drying skincare products and practices.

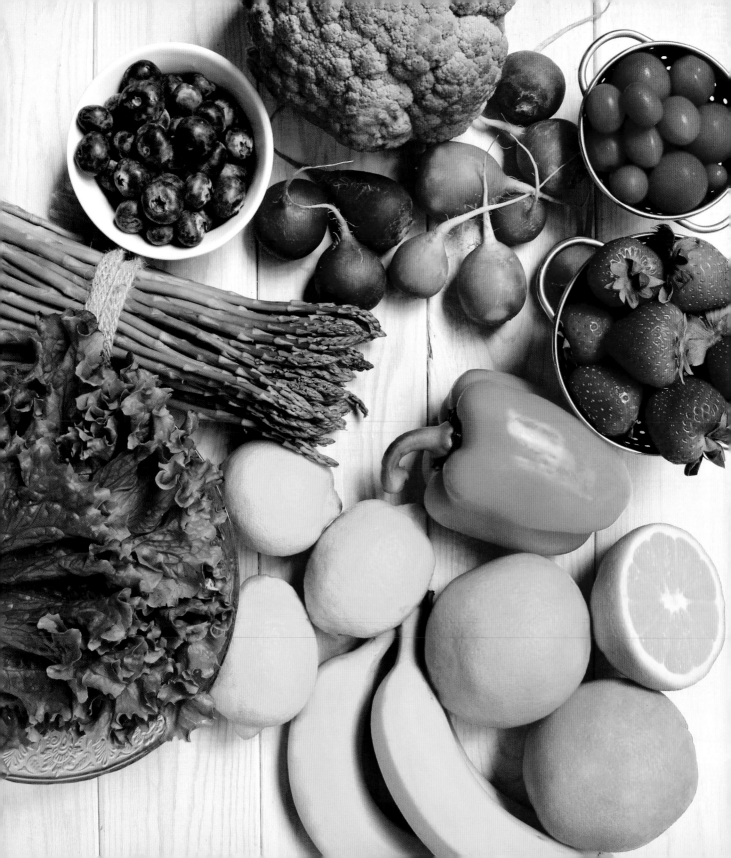

Glowing Skin From Within

• • •

FEED YOUR SKIN THE GLOW-GETTING NUTRIENTS IT'S CRAVING

THE YUMMIEST AND SUREST WAY TO GORGEOUS SKIN

"Feed me!"—Your skin

Can you hear that? It's your skin begging for the nutrients it needs to get its glow on. Because to build healthy skin, we need to provide our bodies with the necessary building blocks. These building blocks are nutrients.

Unfortunately, the modern diet is seriously lacking in quality nutrients. The reason: Around 70 percent of the modern diet is composed of processed foods. These packaged, food-like products are loaded with inferior macronutrients—especially cheap "vegetable" oils and refined, simple carbohydrates like sugar, corn and wheat—and stripped of their life-giving, glow-getting micronutrients (not to mention the fact that they also contain unhealthy artificial colors, preservatives and flavorings, some of which have even been banned in other countries). Yes, even many of those so-called healthy cereals and nutrition bars. These are simply not the foods our bodies were designed to run on, yet alone thrive on. So, is it any wonder our skin is paying the price?

When it comes to feeding your skin the nutrients it's craving, it's a matter of:

1. Making the switch to a real food diet

2. Incorporating each of the glow-getting macronutrients in each meal

3. Seeking out the glow-getting micronutrients

The very first step to getting the proper building blocks for naturally gorgeous skin is simply adopting a real food diet.

Although I say "simply" here, for many people this is really anything but and requires quite a dramatic transformation in both thought and habit. After all, processed foods are everywhere. They're easily accessible and make up the majority of the average person's diet. They're familiar and comfortable, and often comforting. They're sometimes cheaper than whole foods and often more convenient.

But ditching processed foods for real food is without a doubt the most significant change you can make for your health and skin. Fueling your body with nutrient-dense real foods will have you looking great and feeling even better.

REAL FOODS BASICS

EAT REAL FOOD. (Duh!) This means no processed foods and no mystery ingredients. Foods should be in their whole, natural form (or something very close to it). Does this mean you should never, ever have a processed food ever again? No! But it should be an occasional, rare indulgence rather the norm—on the average day, all of your meals and snacks should be recognizable as real food. Trust me when I tell you it's not nearly as difficult as it may now seem, both in regard to prep time and flavor satisfaction. And one day, you'll probably even find yourself looking at [insert name of favorite processed food here] and wondering, "I actually used to put this STUFF in my body!?"

EAT A VARIETY OF REAL FOODS. Carrots are great. And carrots do constitute a "real food." But carrots all day every day? You'd be lacking the macronutrients fat and protein, as well as countless micronutrients. You'd be malnourished and wouldn't survive very long. Not to mention the fact that your skin would likely be orange from all of the beta-carotene—think: Oompa Loompa or *Jersey Shore* cast member. So, switch things up! Eating a diverse range of real foods will help ensure you're getting an array of glow-getting nutrients.

EAT THE RAINBOW. Eat real foods of all different colors to further ensure you're getting a wide variety of beautifying nutrients. Vibrant purple figs, dark green spinach, bright orange sweet potatoes, ruby red tomatoes . . . they all provide your skin with different glow-getting nutrients.

And no, it's not possible to supplement your way to healthy skin! First of all, processed foods are filled with ingredients that are doing irreparable harm and need to be eliminated, not simply compensated for. Second, our bodies were designed to assimilate vitamins and minerals from whole foods, not pills. Vitamins and minerals in supplements are often synthetic forms of the nutrients. This does not mean that they can't remedy deficiencies, but it is always best to first obtain nutrients in their natural form through diet. Furthermore, many nutrients work in synergy with each other and come packaged together in real foods (because Mother Nature is one smart lady), increasing their benefit.

AT THE GROCERY STORE, STEER CLEAR OF THE CENTER AISLES!

This is where all the processed foods are shelved. Fresh produce, meat, dairy, eggs and seafood are all along the periphery of the store. Of course, you'll need to venture into these aisles to buy certain real food staples, such as shredded coconut, olive oil, nuts and tomato paste. But when you do so, stick to your mission! Grab what you need and don't get distracted by those colorful boxes with mile-long ingredient lists.

Now let's get into the nitty-gritty and look at which specific nutrients your skin is craving.

We need to go beyond real food and look at the macronutrients and micronutrients required to build, protect and repair the skin.

MACRONUTRIENTS

Meet your macronutrients: protein, fat and carbohydrate. Unfortunately, we receive a lot of mixed messages about this trio. Do any of these look familiar?

CUT ALL CARBS TO LOSE WEIGHT AND BE HEALTHY!

A COMPLETELY PLANT-BASED, HIGH-CARB DIET IS BEST!

ANIMAL PROTEIN WILL KILL YOU!

EAT ALL THE ANIMALS, JUST LIKE OUR CAVEMAN ANCESTORS!

FAT IS YOUR ENEMY; KEEP IT FAR, FAR AWAY!

A HIGH-FAT DIET KEEPS YOU FEELING FULL AND THIN!

It's downright confusing, and can cause people to knowingly eliminate an entire macronutrient group from their diet. But doing so is a recipe for disaster. Humans require proteins, fats and carbohydrates to maintain vibrant health and build beautiful skin. That being said, quality is of the utmost importance when it comes to the macronutrients—eliminating the skin-sacrificing sources and increasing the glow-getting sources is of equal importance.

PROTEIN

The word *protein* is actually derived from the ancient Greek root meaning "of first importance," which is a clue into just how important this macronutrient is for our health. During digestion, proteins are broken down into amino acids, which are used to build and repair cells. This is especially important for the skin, which sheds and regenerates constantly, with an entirely new layer created each month. Our bodies and skin age prematurely without adequate dietary protein—cells cannot repair and regenerate themselves quickly enough, leading to wrinkling and poor wound healing.

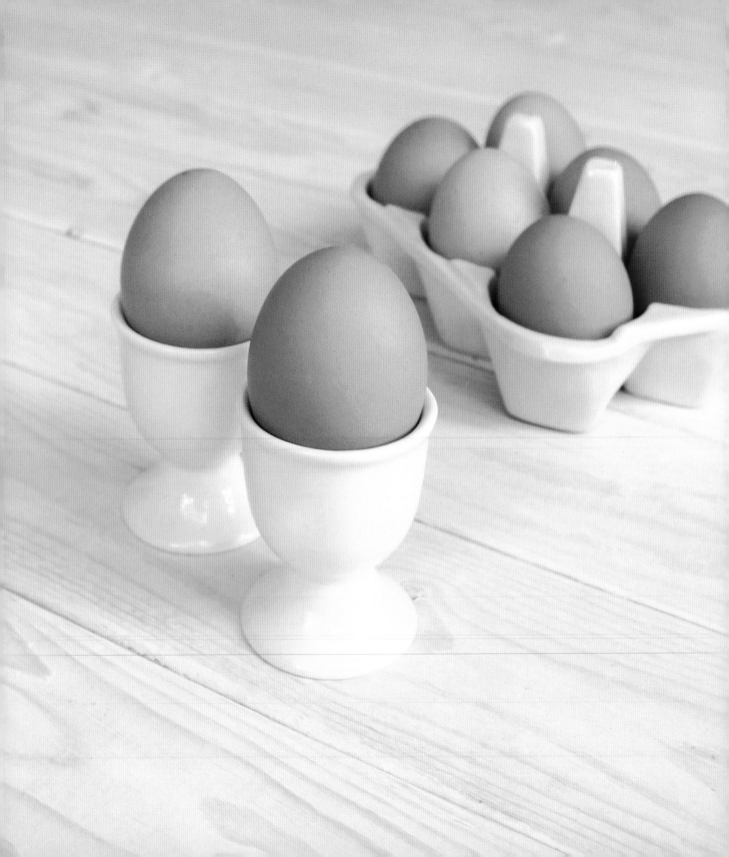

Our bodies make eleven of the twenty amino acids that are essential to life, meaning we must get the remaining nine amino acids through diet. Proteins that contain these nine essential amino acids are called complete proteins. Since protein cannot be stored in our bodies, we need to make sure we're getting adequate amounts of protein daily, ideally with each meal.

GLOW-GETTING SOURCES OF PROTEIN

- Grass-fed beef*
- Pasture-raised poultry*
- Pasture-raised eggs*
- Wild-caught fish*
- Buckwheat*
- Quinoa*
- Chia seeds*
- Legumes
- Other nuts and seeds

*Complete proteins

SKIN-SACRIFICING SOURCES OF PROTEIN

- Conventional beef produced in factory farms
- Conventional poultry produced in factory farms
- Unfermented soy
- Low- or nonfat dairy products

WHY THE EMPHASIS ON GRASS-FED AND PASTURE-RAISED ANIMAL PRODUCTS?

Animal proteins are the best dietary sources of vitamins A, D and K_2, as well as the only dietary source of B_{12}, each of which you'll soon learn is critical for skin health. But for health, environmental and ethical reasons, it's important to choose quality animal proteins. Sadly, most of the beef, chicken, dairy and eggs found in grocery stores today come from factory farms where animals are treated extremely unethically. In these facilities, chickens and cows are loaded with antibiotics and fed an unnatural diet. Cows are also given hormones to grow faster or produce more milk. These antibiotics and hormones make their way onto our dinner plates and are a significant cause for concern. On the other hand, meat, dairy and eggs from animals allowed to roam on pasture and eat their natural diet are often proudly raised by ethical farmers who do not use antibiotics or hormones. And they're nutritionally superior, too:

- Grass-fed beef contains greater amounts of anti-inflammatory omega-3 essential fatty acids as well as the glow-getting vitamins A, C, E and B_{12}.
- Eggs from pasture-raised hens contain more of the glow-getting vitamins A and E as well as more anti-inflammatory, skin-soothing omega-3 fatty acids.
- Raw grass-fed dairy products are rich in vitamins A, D and K_2. Raw dairy also contains lactase, the enzyme needed to digest lactose. Pasteurization kills lactase, which is why so many people have such a difficult time digesting dairy.

SKIN-LOVING SUPERFOOD SPOTLIGHT: GELATIN

This protein packed superfood helps smooth skin from the inside out.

Gelatin is essentially cooked collagen, which you'll recall is a protein found in the dermis that keeps the skin looking smooth and youthful. While collagen is key to a youthful complexion, it's worthless in skincare products—the molecules are too large to be absorbed by the skin! But dietary collagen is a different story.

As we get older, collagen synthesis decreases and existing collagen fibers become weak, causing the skin to lose elasticity. By supplementing with gelatin in either its whole form or as collagen peptides, you're giving your body the exact amino acids it needs to help maintain and restore skin elasticity. Bonus: Gelatin helps heal the gut lining, support bone and joint health, aids digestion and is rich in skin-supporting minerals.

Bone broth is a fantastic source of gelatin that you can make at home. You can also purchase high-quality supplemental gelatin and collagen peptides sourced from grass-fed cows. I start each day with a tablespoon of collagen peptides to accompany my breakfast and add them to my smoothies for added protein and skin-loving goodness.

CARBOHYDRATES

Carbohydrates provide the body with a critical source of energy: glucose. This energy allows cells to carry out all of their vital processes. Glow-getting carbohydrates also help regulate fat and protein metabolism and provide the body with protective vitamins, minerals and antioxidants. Plus, the fiber and nutrients in glow-getting carbohydrates help the body to process the natural sugars they contain. (Remember: Mother Nature knows what she's doing.)

The majority of our dietary carbohydrates should be coming from whole fruits and vegetables, and a smaller amount from unrefined, gluten-free grains, legumes and natural sweeteners.

GLOW-GETTING SOURCES OF CARBOHYDRATES

- Fruits
- Vegetables
- Gluten-free grains (in moderation), such as quinoa, buckwheat, oats, amaranth and rice
- Legumes (in moderation)
- Natural sweeteners (in moderation), such as raw honey, 100% pure blackstrap molasses, coconut sugar and maple syrup

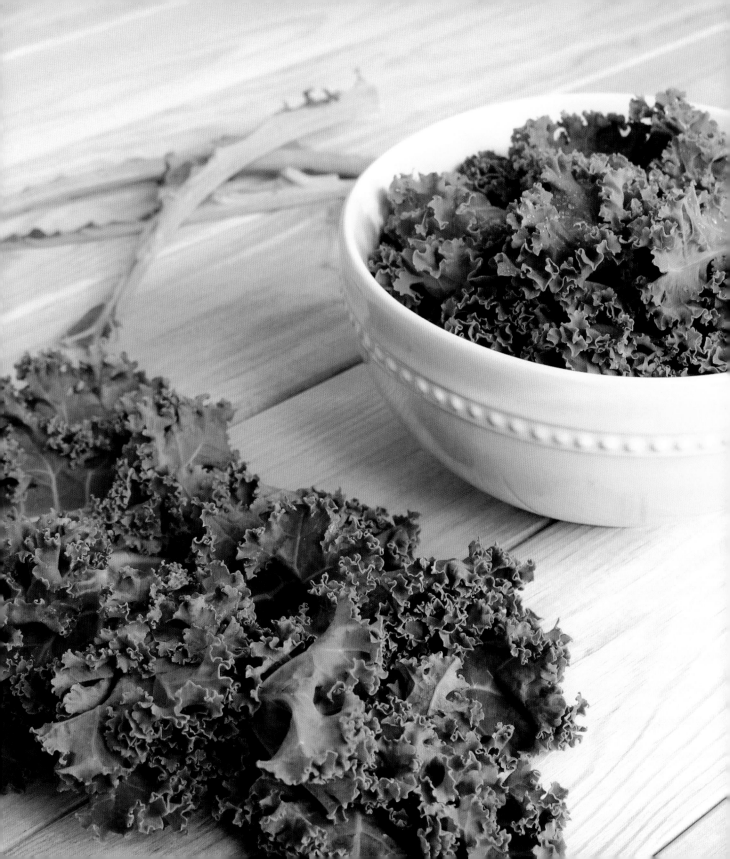

Sugar and refined, simple carbohydrates contribute to each of the internal imbalances that undermine skin health, so expect to read a lot more about them in the pages to come! As often as possible, it is best to avoid these skin-sacrificing sources of carbohydrates.

SKIN-SACRIFICING SOURCES OF CARBOHYDRATES

- Cane sugar

- High-fructose corn syrup

- The gluten-containing grains wheat, barley, rye and triticale (a rye/wheat hybrid)

- Refined corn

WHAT'S THE DEAL WITH GLUTEN?

Ah, gluten: the little protein found in wheat that has had everyone and their grandma going gaga. Well, unfortunately, the rumors seem to be true. Numerous studies and an unending amount of anecdotal evidence suggest that gluten is unhealthy, even for those individuals without an allergy or intolerance. This is likely due to the fact that gluten damages the gut lining, causing chronic inflammation and increasing the permeability of the intestines. We'll get into the details a bit more later, but for now know that the gluten-free phenomena isn't just some crunchy woo-woo or a passing fad, and that gluten-containing grains are best to be avoided.

Honestly, removing gluten from your diet is a lot easier than it seems at first. In fact, if you're sticking to a real food diet, it's quite simple since the majority of gluten-containing foods are processed (cereals, crackers, pasta, bread, etc.). If anything, avoiding gluten is just another great reason to focus on real foods.

SKIN-LOVING SUPERFOOD SPOTLIGHT: LEAFY GREENS

Leafy greens continue to reign supreme over all the veggies and are one glow-getting source of carbs I suggest fitting into your diet every single day. They're jam-packed with skin-protecting antioxidants as well as fiber, folic acid, vitamin C, potassium and magnesium.

The most nutrient-dense greens include cabbage, kale, dandelion greens, romaine lettuce, spinach, mustard greens, turnip greens, collard greens and Swiss chard. Iceberg lettuce, on the other hand, contains very few nutrients.

If you don't quite have a taste for greens, sneak them in via a delicious smoothie! This also makes them easier to digest, which can be an issue for some. And not only are frozen organic greens much cheaper than their fresh counterparts, but they're also virtually tasteless when added to a smoothie. Go ahead and see for yourself! And if you're looking for a good recipe, check out my Go-to Green Smoothie (page 100).

FAT

Fat is a vital nutrient, not a monster! It provides the body with a concentrated source of energy and is a primary component of cell membranes, making it absolutely critical for healthy skin. It also keeps skin supple and moisturized, is imperative for the digestion of cell-building protein, is key in the body's healing process and is necessary for the absorption of the fat-soluble vitamins A, D, E and K, each of which is vital for skin health.

But not all fats are created equally! Some nourish the skin while others inflame it.

SATURATED FATS make up at least 50 percent of cell membranes, which is why they are necessary for proper cell structure and function. Saturated fats are also a key ingredient for building healthy hormones, protecting the liver from toxins and boosting the immune system.

Okay, let's address the elephant in the room: Saturated fat has a bad reputation! It has been wrongly accused of causing heart disease since the mid-1900s. But this was largely based on grossly misinterpreted studies and did not take other factors into consideration (the increased consumption of processed carbohydrates, sugar or refined and hydrogenated plant oils). Study upon study has debunked the connection between saturated fat and heart disease, yet the story continued to stick. In recent years, saturated fat has become quite the comeback kid, with grass-fed beef, butter, eggs and coconut oil reclaiming their rightful place in the kitchen.

Since saturated fats have a stable molecular structure, they are ideal for high-heat cooking, do not go rancid easily and are solid or semisolid at room temperature.

MONOUNSATURATED FATS are the easy ones of the bunch—they are widely accepted as healthy.

These relatively stable fats may be used for low-temperature cooking, do not go rancid very easily and are liquid at room temperature. Always choose cold-pressed and/or extra-virgin sources of monounsaturated oils, and choose products in dark glass bottles, which will help protect these more fragile fatty acids.

POLYUNSATURATED FATS can be subdivided into omega-3 (alpha-linolenic acid) and omega-6 (linoleic acid) fatty acids. This duo is known as the essential fatty acids since our bodies can't produce them and they must be obtained from our diet. That being said, we don't need much of them for optimal health—they should constitute just around 4 percent of our daily caloric intake. Although we ought to be consuming about the same amounts of these fatty acids, the average person is getting ten to twenty times more omega-6 fatty acids than omega-3s, thanks to the widespread use of cheap "vegetable" oils in processed foods. This promotes skin-sabotaging inflammation, as we will soon discuss in greater detail. For this reason, omega-3 polyunsaturated fatty acids should be sought out, while omega-6 polyunsaturated fatty acids should be reduced. And the cheap "vegetable" oils— canola, sunflower, safflower, soybean, corn and cottonseed oil—should never be touched!

Since polyunsaturated fats are extremely unstable and go rancid quite easily, they should never be used for cooking or heated in any way, and should be refrigerated and stored in dark containers.

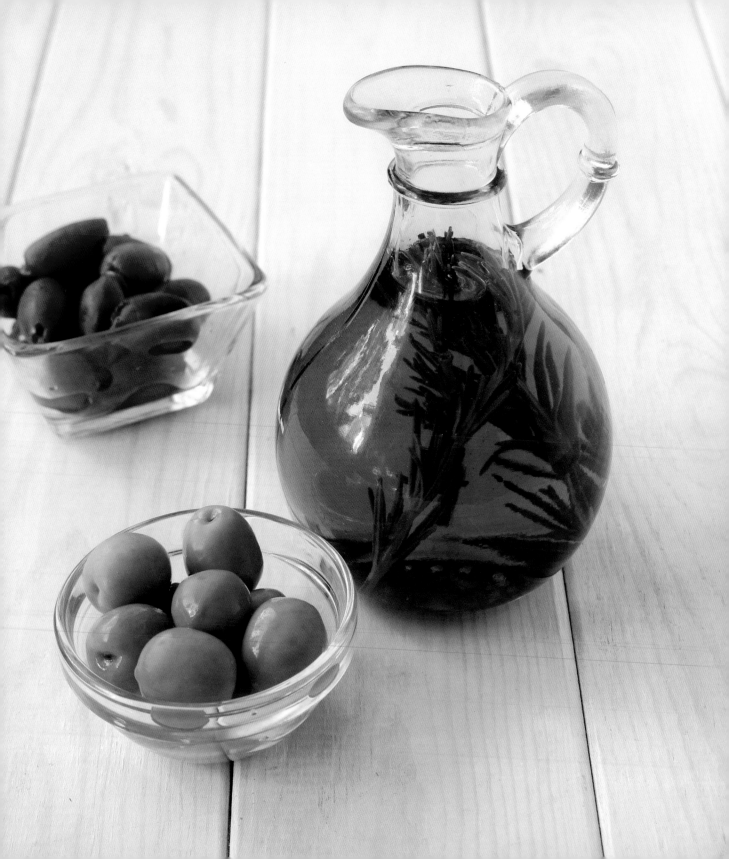

TRANS FATS are the fake fats to avoid like the plague. Trans fats are a by-product of hydrogenation, a process that solidifies oil that would otherwise be liquid at room temperature by forcing hydrogen atoms into the oil's structure, using a chemical catalyst. Once upon a time, food chemists called them plastic oils (yummy). Hydrogenation was invented to extend the shelf life of fragile, polyunsaturated "vegetable" oils, as well as the shelf life of processed foods containing these oils. While this may sound like a good thing, it's really anything but. The altered chemical structure of the oil causes chronic inflammation and an increased risk of insulin resistance. Not only does this spell B-I-G T-R-O-U-B-L-E for your skin, the Harvard School of Public Health reports that every 2 percent increase in daily calories from trans fats increases risk of coronary heart disease by a whopping 23 percent! I truly believe that this is one ingredient that should not be consumed in any quantity, no matter how small.

GLOW-GETTING SOURCES OF FAT

- Saturated fats
  - Coconut and coconut oil
  - Grass-fed meat
  - Full-fat, grass-fed raw or organic dairy products
  - Pasture-raised eggs
  - Sustainably sourced red palm
- Monounsaturated fats
  - Avocados and avocado oil
  - Olives and olive oil
  - Almonds
  - Hazelnuts
  - Macadamia nuts
- Polyunsaturated fats
  - Wild-caught fish
  - Walnuts
  - Wheat germ
  - Flaxseeds
  - Hemp seeds
  - Pumpkin seeds

SKIN-SABOTAGING SOURCES OF FATS

- "Vegetable" oils, including canola, sunflower, safflower, soybean, corn and cottonseed oils
- Nonorganic dairy products
- Hydrogenated oils

SHOULDN'T DAIRY BE AVOIDED?

You've likely heard it suggested to avoid dairy if you have acne, and I generally agree with this—as will be explained in more detail later, dairy can exacerbate acne by stimulating hormones that increase sebum production. And many people are intolerant to dairy, in which case it should also be avoided, since food intolerances are a major source of skin-irritating inflammation.

But this is really not a simple question to answer as there is a huge difference between the grain-fed dairy that you'll find in most grocery stores and grass-fed raw or organic dairy. Grain-fed dairy is nutritionally deficient, contains synthetic antibiotics and hormones (commonly used in factory farm operations), and has been stripped of lactase, the enzyme required to digest lactose (the process of pasteurization kills lactase along with potentially harmful pathogens). Grass-fed dairy is a rich source of the glow-getting vitamins A, D, E and K_2, and organic dairy is produced without the use of synthetic antibiotics and hormones. Raw dairy is special since it has not been pasteurized—a process that really only became necessary with the advent of unsanitary factory farms—and so still contains lactase, making it much easier to digest. For these reasons, many consider grass-fed raw and organic dairy to actually be very nutritious, and a number of studies support this.

There's also a concern of casein, a protein in dairy products that has been linked to cancer. But what's often missing from this conversation is whey, another protein found in dairy that has been found to have cancer-fighting properties.

My personal opinion? If you have acne, a food intolerance to dairy or you're not able to buy quality, grass-fed raw or organic dairy products, dairy shouldn't be on the menu—it is not critical for good health and there are plenty of other sources of the fat-soluble vitamins. But otherwise, grass-fed raw and organic dairy can be very nourishing to the body and skin.

SKIN-LOVING SUPERFOOD SPOTLIGHT: COCONUT OIL

Everyone's gone cuckoo for coconut recently, and for good reason. Coconut oil is unique because it is rich in medium-chain triglycerides (MCTs), which do not require bile acids for digestion but are instead directly shunted to the liver. This means that they are immediately converted to energy and not readily stored as fat. A number of studies have shown that MCTs can even boost metabolism—one found that 1 to 2 tablespoons (15 to 30 ml) of coconut oil a day increased the daily energy expenditure of participants by an average of 120 calories.

Lauric acid is one of the most notable MCTs in coconut oil. Lauric acid is inherently antibacterial as well as a precursor to an even more powerful antimicrobial agent that is synthesized in the digestive tract, and as such helps boost the immune system and fight unhealthy microbes in the gut. For reasons we will soon learn, this is extremely beneficial to the skin.

Unrefined coconut oil maintains a slightly sweet coconut taste, whereas refined coconut oil has virtually no taste. Both are a staple in my kitchen, with unrefined coconut oil going into smoothies and being used for baking and refined coconut oil being used primarily for cooking.

Each macronutrient should be included in every meal, since this trio plays extremely well together.

Carbohydrates provide the body with its preferred source of fuel, while protein pulls that fuel source into the cells so the body can use it for energy. Healthy fats and protein keep you feeling full and satiated while slowing the absorption of glucose into the bloodstream (this is very important for blood sugar balance, and will be discussed in more detail in the next section).

How much of each macronutrient we should be consuming varies, since we're biologically unique individuals. I am a big believer in listening to your body and finding a balance that works best for you rather than listening to dietary dogma and adhering to abstract numbers, which don't take biological individuality into account. However, if you're just beginning to find the best balance of macronutrients for your body, start by eating 30 percent of your daily caloric intake from fat, 30 percent from protein and 40 percent from carbohydrates—this is a good ratio for keeping blood sugar levels steady. Take note of how your body feels with your food journal (see page 13) and adjust accordingly.

WATER: THE "FOURTH MACRONUTRIENT"?

Some consider water to be a macronutrient right alongside protein, carbohydrate and fat. Its importance is certainly undeniable—we can go weeks without food but only days without water.

Water makes up 55 to 60 percent of our bodies and around 65 percent of our skin. It is responsible for a whole bunch of vital processes, from flushing toxins to transporting nutrients within cells, and is also vital to the body's natural healing processes. Each of these processes is critical to the health of the skin. And, of course, water also helps keep the skin hydrated, giving it a softer tone and more youthful appearance.

But many of us do not get nearly as much water as our bodies require. Here's a simple way to calculate how many ounces of water you should be drinking daily:

YOUR BODY WEIGHT ÷ 2 = DAILY MINIMUM H_2O INTAKE IN OZ*

Now, you can't just consider all fluids/drinks "water"—not all fluid is hydrating! In fact, many are dehydrating. These are called diuretics. Common diuretics include coffee, tea (some herbals excluded) and juice. So, let's adjust this equation, taking diuretics into consideration:

[OZ OF DIURETICS × 1.5] + [YOUR BODY WEIGHT ÷ 2] = DAILY MINIMUM H_2O INTAKE IN OZ*

*Do not exceed 100 ounces (3 L) of water a day.

Of course, these formulas are not absolute—they do not take such factors as physical activity (the more you sweat, the more you will need to hydrate) or physical conditions (pregnant women, for example, require more water) into account. So, consider the final number to be a ballpark figure rather than fixed.

It's very important to hydrate slowly and consistently throughout the day—chugging a large amount of water at one time can actually flush out electrolytes and dehydrate the body since water depends on electrolytes for proper absorption. Ironic, right?

MICRONUTRIENTS

If you're following the real foods basics outlined at the beginning of this chapter and incorporating glow-getting sources of each macronutrient in your diet, you're well on your way to ensuring your skin is receiving a wide range of beautifying micronutrients: vitamins and minerals. From vitamin A to zinc, these micronutrients are critical to maintaining healthy, glowing skin.

VITAMIN A: This fat-soluble antioxidant vitamin neutralizes free radicals, protecting skin from the damaging effects of pollution and the sun. It is also critical for cellular turnover and regeneration, stimulating new cell growth while also supporting the structural integrity of cells. But it is necessary to understand the difference between preformed vitamin A (retinol) and provitamin A: Preformed vitamin A is readily available for the body to use, whereas the body must convert provitamin A to a usable form of vitamin A, and this conversion does not typically yield a significant amount.

- **Sources of preformed vitamin A:** cod liver oil, egg yolks, liver, raw grass-fed dairy, red meat
- **Sources of provitamin A:** asparagus, broccoli, Brussels sprouts, butternut squash, cantaloupe, carrots, cherries, kale, mangoes, papayas, peaches, pumpkin, sweet potatoes, watermelon, winter squash, yams

VITAMIN B$_2$ (RIBOFLAVIN): This B vitamin is necessary for normal cell growth and helps cells utilize oxygen most efficiently. New research has also shown that vitamin B$_2$ has an antioxidant effect, protecting cells from damaging free radicals.

- **Sources of vitamin B$_2$:** asparagus, brewer's yeast, broccoli, eggs, liver, mackerel, peas, spinach, sunflower seeds, trout

VITAMIN B$_3$ (NIACIN): Vitamin B$_3$ is a key player in DNA repair, keeping cells healthy. It is particularly important to the skin, which experiences quick cell turnover.

- **Sources of vitamin B$_3$:** avocados, dates, eggs, figs, halibut, liver, poultry, prunes, salmon

VITAMIN B$_5$ (PANTOTHENIC ACID): Vitamin B$_5$ has earned itself the nickname "the antistress vitamin" since it supports the adrenal glands, helping to counteract emotional and physical stress on the body. Because of this, it is thought to help prevent premature aging and wrinkle formation.

- **Sources of vitamin B$_5$:** avocados, cauliflower, chicken, egg yolks, fish, liver, mushrooms, peanuts, sweet potatoes

VITAMIN B$_6$ (PYRIDOXINE): Vitamin B$_6$ is critical for protein metabolism, helping transport those cell-building, glow-getting amino acids into cells. It also supports the immune system and is critical for the production and proper functioning of DNA.

- **Sources of vitamin B$_6$:** butternut squash, egg yolks, fish, liver, peanuts, poultry, walnuts

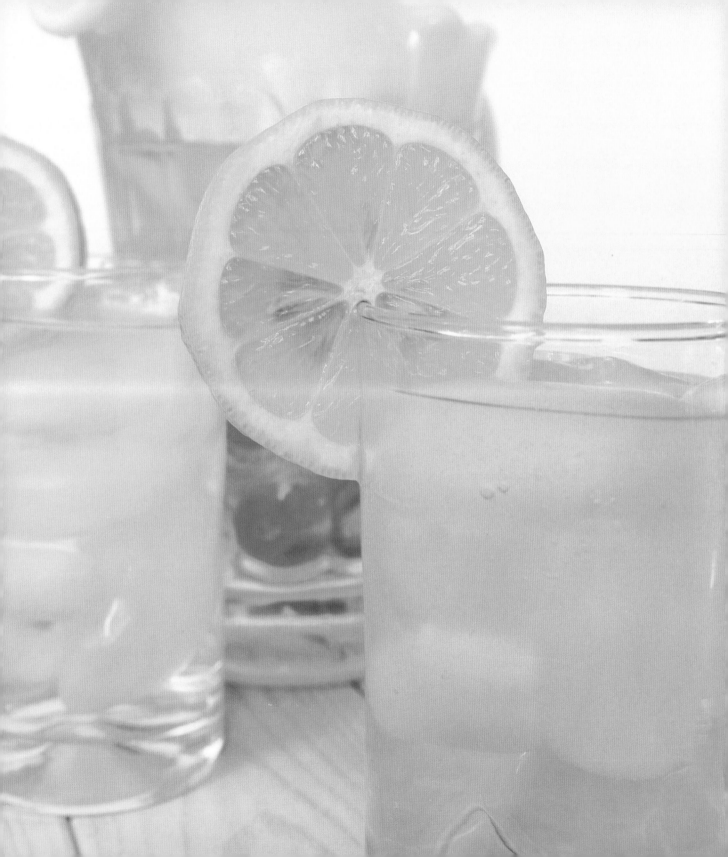

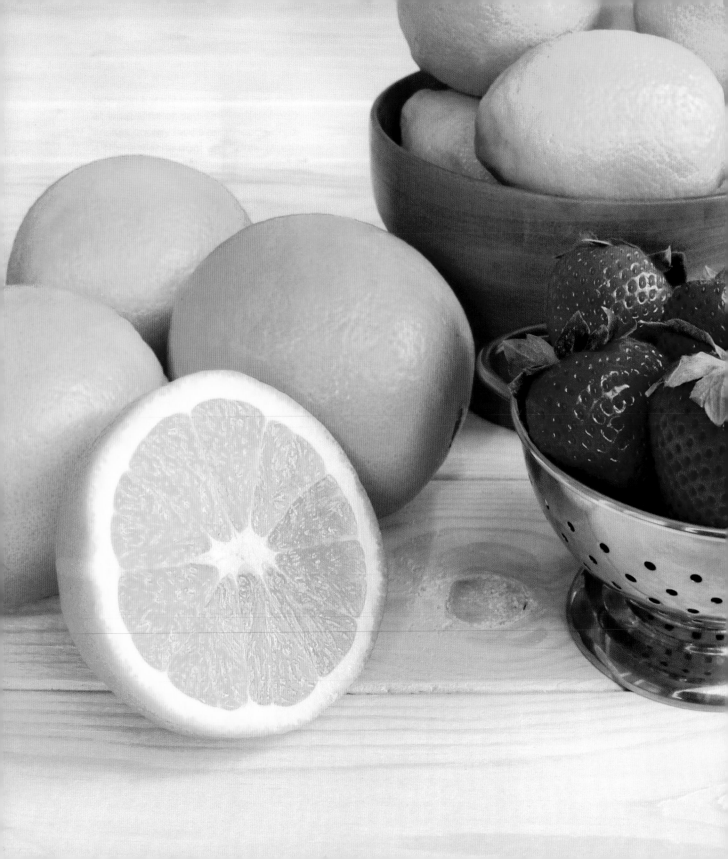

VITAMIN B$_7$ (BIOTIN): This B vitamin is critical for fat metabolism, making it key for the formation of new tissue. Since skin cells are shed and regenerated very quickly, biotin plays a key role in skin health. For this reason, biotin is often used to support the skin of those suffering from dermatitis and eczema.

- **Sources of vitamin B$_7$:** almonds, cabbage, egg yolks, liver, onions, romaine lettuce, Swiss chard, walnuts

NOTE: The best source of vitamin B$_7$ is the healthy gut flora housed in our very own GI tracts, which is one of the chief reasons why it's so important to keep our guts healthy!

VITAMIN B$_9$ (FOLATE): This B vitamin is critical for healthy skin since it plays a key role in cell division and growth, which the skin cells experience constantly and rapidly.

- **Sources of vitamin B$_9$:** asparagus, avocados, beet greens, chard, kale, spinach

NOTE: Folic acid is the synthetic form of folate found in many supplements. It is advised to seek out folate instead of folic acid.

VITAMIN B$_{12}$ (COBALAMIN): Nicknamed "the longevity vitamin" and "the energy vitamin," vitamin B$_{12}$ is critical for healthy energy use and metabolism.

- **Sources of vitamin B$_{12}$:** organ meats, poultry, red meat

NOTE: Vegetarians must take care to supplement with vitamin B$_{12}$ since animal proteins are the most significant dietary sources of this crucial vitamin.

VITAMIN C: A potent antioxidant, this free radical fighter is well known for boosting the immune system. It is also a necessary precursor for both collagen and elastin, keeping skin smooth and elastic. It also helps wounds heal more quickly and maintain healthy blood vessels.

- **Sources of vitamin C:** asparagus, bell peppers, broccoli, Brussels sprouts, butternut squash, citrus fruits, guavas, kale, kiwis, spinach, tomatoes

COPPER: This mineral works with vitamin C to form collagen and helps support the healing process of skin tissue.

- **Sources of copper:** almonds, Brazil nuts, buckwheat, hazelnuts, liver, mushrooms, pecans, prunes, shellfish, walnuts

NOTE: Few people are deficient in copper. On the contrary, copper toxicity is more of a concern. So, while this mineral plays a key role in the body and skin health, know that you likely consume enough of it naturally and do not need to seek it out in your diet or through supplementation.

VITAMIN D: "The sunshine vitamin" is absolutely critical for the body's immune system, including the skin's natural defenses. As with vitamin A, there are two different forms of vitamin D. Vitamin D_3 is created naturally in the skin and is considered by some researchers to be the only active form of vitamin D. Since it is formed when a specific type of cholesterol in our skin interacts with sunlight and cholesterol is only found in animals, vitamin D_3 can only be obtained through diet from animal products (though there are some vegan supplements options for D_3). Small amounts of vitamin D_2 is found in certain plants, though it is not believed to have the same effects on the body as natural vitamin D_3.

- **Sources of vitamin D_3:** The sun! Cod liver oil, egg yolks, grass-fed dairy products, herring, mackerel, salmon and sardines are good dietary sources of this critical vitamin.

VITAMIN E: This fat-soluble antioxidant is great at protecting fats in the body from oxidation, a process that creates free radicals and systemic inflammation and is a likely contributor to breakouts. For this reason, vitamin E helps maintain the integrity of cell membranes, which are comprised mostly of lipids. This powerful vitamin also helps wounds and scars heal more quickly.

- **Sources of vitamin E:** almonds, asparagus, avocados, beet greens, collard greens, mangoes, pumpkin, red bell peppers, spinach, sunflower seeds

IRON: Iron is a key player in the cytochrome system, which protects tissues and cells from free radical damage. This helps keep cells and skin healthy and young.

- **Sources of iron:** lentils, liver, mussels, oysters, poultry, red meat, sardines, spinach

VITAMIN K_1: This fat-soluble vitamin is necessary for the formation of certain proteins that maintain healthy skin cells. Recent research also indicates that it may help maintain skin elasticity and therefore prevent premature aging.

- **Sources of vitamin K_1:** collard greens, kale, spinach

VITAMIN K₂: This fat-soluble vitamin shuttles calcium to where it belongs, such as in the bones and teeth, and prevents it from depositing where it does not belong. For this reason, it prevents the calcification of our skin's collagen and elastin, which would cause these fibers to harden and contribute to premature aging of the skin.

- **Sources of vitamin K₂:** grass-fed dairy products, egg yolks, liver, natto, sauerkraut

> **NOTE:** This vitamin is produced in the large intestine by the healthy gut flora—just one of the many reasons a diverse and robust gut microbiome is so important!

MAGNESIUM: This vital mineral increases cell growth and is a cofactor in collagen production. It also helps reduce inflammation and keep hormones balanced. Last but not least, magnesium helps facilitate the transfer of other nutrients across cell membranes, allowing skin cells to benefit from all of the other glow-getting nutrients!

- **Sources of magnesium:** almonds, avocados, kale, pecans, spinach, sunflower seeds

MANGANESE: This mineral activates the enzymes that allow the body to use some very important other beauty-boosting micronutrients, such as vitamin B₁, biotin and vitamin C. It's also important for protein digestion, which is imperative for building healthy skin cells.

- **Sources of manganese:** chickpeas, egg yolks, kale, potatoes, spinach

SELENIUM: This mineral has an antioxidant effect on cells, working in sync with vitamin E to protect the lipids in cell membranes from oxidation. It is also critical for proper thyroid functioning.

- **Sources of selenium:** Brazil nuts, eggs, grass-fed beef, halibut, liver, molasses, poultry, sardines, spinach, tuna

SILICA: This mineral is a key component of collagen, keeping the skin strong and firm.

- **Sources of silica:** asparagus, celery, chickpeas, cucumbers, green beans, leeks, mangoes, onions, radishes, rhubarb, strawberries

SULFUR: This mineral is necessary for collagen production as well as for the synthesis of glutathione, one of the most powerful and important antioxidants in the body. High levels of glutathione help prevent free radical damage, which accelerates skin aging.

- **Sources of sulfur:** asparagus, broccoli, Brussels sprouts, eggs, fish, garlic, grass-fed beef, grass-fed dairy, kale, onions, poultry, radishes

ZINC: This vital mineral aids cell repair and regeneration and supports the production of elastin. Zinc also plays an important anti-inflammatory role in the skin's immune system, which is why it's especially helpful for those suffering from inflammatory skin conditions, such as acne, eczema and rosacea.

- **Sources of zinc:** cacao, cashews, chia seeds, chickpeas, egg yolks, grass-fed beef, liver, oysters, poultry, pumpkin seeds, quinoa

NOTE: Studies have found individuals with acne tend to have lower levels of zinc than do individuals without acne, and that zinc levels and the severity of acne are inversely proportional (in other words, the lower the zinc, the more severe the acne). It's similarly been suggested that people with eczema are zinc deficient. Studies have also found zinc helpful in reducing the severity of rosacea.

SWITCH YOUR SALT FOR EXTRA SKIN-LOVING GOODNESS!

Whereas refined table salt is stripped of much of its natural mineral content, unrefined sea salt contains dozens of minerals the skin loves. Celtic sea salt and pink Himalayan sea salt are my two personal favorites. The rule of thumb: Avoid white salt. Do keep in mind, however, that unrefined sea salt is not iodized—iodine is an important mineral that is necessary for normal thyroid function, which is why it is added to most refined table salt. So, you will need to seek out iodine from other food sources or supplement with kelp, a fantastic source of iodine.

Each meal is an opportunity to nourish your skin from within.

Eliminating processed, refined foods from your diet and replacing them with real, whole foods is undoubtedly the most profound change you can make for your skin. Once you're following the real foods basics and including the appropriate types of each macronutrient at each meal, you'll realize that nourishing your skin from within is actually quite simple! Because within the macronutrients, you'll find all of the glow-getting micronutrients from vitamin A to zinc—you won't even need to search them out.

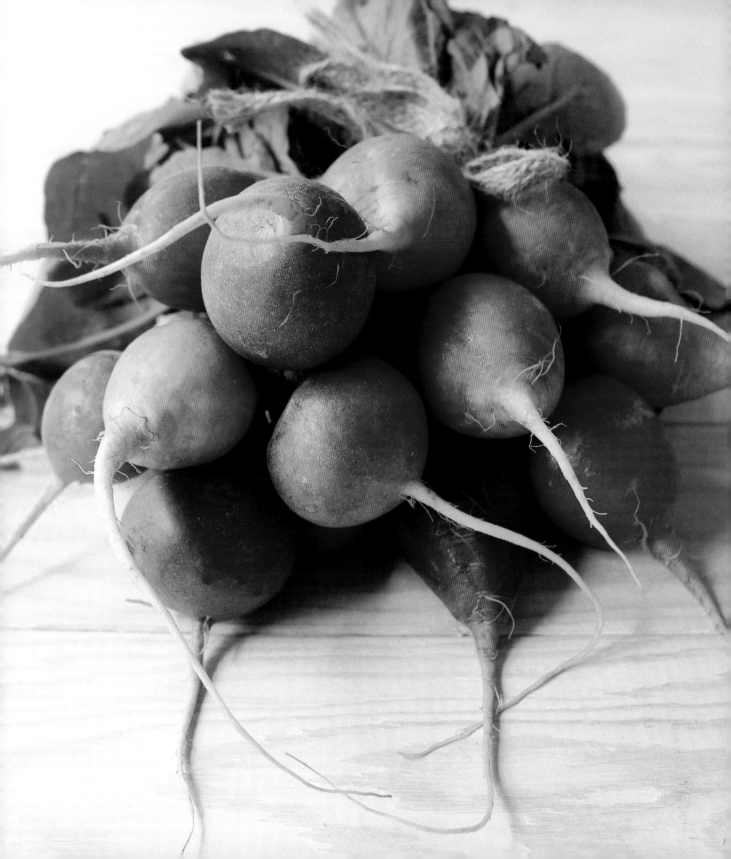

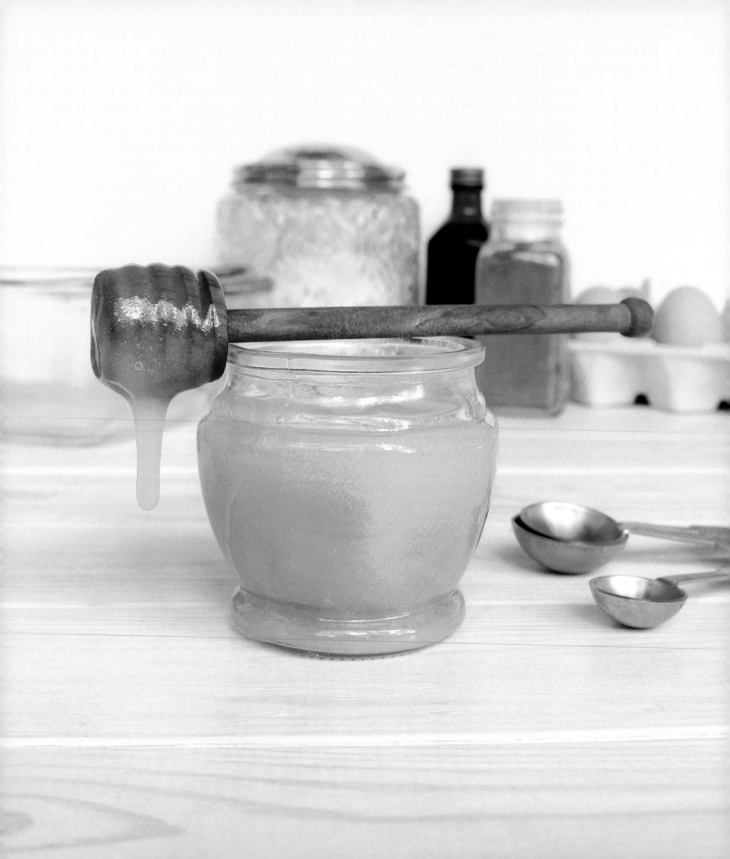

GET OFF THE SKIN-SACRIFICING BLOOD SUGAR ROLLER COASTER

YOUR SKIN IS GETTING WHIPLASH

The majority of us are riding a blood sugar roller coaster, with our skin suffering the consequences.

Sugar and simple carbohydrates, such as corn and wheat flour, are the hallmark of the modern diet. These are not quality sources of fuel for the body and send it on an unending cycle of blood sugar spikes and crashes. But even if you've cut down on sugar and simple carbohydrates, a diet excessively high in healthy carbohydrates can still cause elevated and erratic blood sugar levels. Breakouts, flare-ups and premature skin aging can result, along with weight gain, fatigue, brain fog, midafternoon crashes and "hanger."

Whenever the body detects elevated blood sugar levels, the pancreas is signaled to release insulin, the hormone in charge of shuttling glucose into cells to be used as energy, which brings blood sugar levels back down. This is a natural and necessary process. But over time, excessively high blood sugar levels and the subsequent release of insulin can cause cells to become insulin resistant—cells' resistance to insulin means the glucose remains in the blood (this state of insulin resistance and high blood sugar levels is known as prediabetes). When glucose remains in the bloodstream, a natural process called glycation is accelerated. Glycation is when glucose attaches to proteins in the body—including collagen and elastin—making them rigid. Regular protein versus glycated protein is like a slice of freshly baked bread versus burnt toast—the fresh bread is soft and pliable but the burnt toast will snap right in half. These rigid proteins are called advanced glycation end products (AGEs). AGEs is an incredibly appropriate acronym since these rigid proteins cause premature aging of both the skin and body. Stiff collagen and elastin translates to saggy skin and wrinkles. Perhaps even more concerning than an aging complexion is the fact that AGEs are behind a number of age-related degenerative diseases, such as atherosclerosis, macular degeneration and Alzheimer's.

Elevated and erratic blood sugar levels also impact the skin by triggering each of the other internal imbalances behind most common skin issues:

SUGAR DEPLETES GLOW-GETTING MICRONUTRIENTS. The stress experienced by the body in response to elevated blood sugar levels depletes B vitamins, vitamin C and mineral stores, which skin cells need to generate energy, defend and repair themselves.

SUGAR PROMOTES SKIN-IRRITATING INFLAMMATION. Although insulin is natural and very necessary, high levels—which we experience after eating a sugary food or meal—are extremely inflammatory. AGEs also trigger an inflammatory reaction from the body.

SUGAR HARMS THE GUT. Sugars feed the bad bacteria that are naturally found in the gut, which can then overpower the good gut bacteria. This can lead to a host of digestive issues and gut-related disorders, which we will learn greatly affect the skin.

SUGAR PROMPTS HORMONE IMBALANCES. Increased insulin levels can overstimulate the other hormones. It can cause increased testosterone levels, for example, which stimulates oil gland production, promoting acne. Sugar also taxes the liver, which is key to detoxing excess, used and synthetic hormones to maintain the proper balance.

When it comes to getting off the skin-sacrificing blood sugar roller coaster, it's a matter of:

1. Eliminating sugar and refined, simple carbohydrates from the diet

2. Balancing carbohydrates with adequate protein and fat

3. Using natural, unprocessed sweeteners for a little extra sweetness

Let's be clear: Carbohydrates are not the problem. Certain refined, simple carbohydrates are.

These include:

• Sugar

• Wheat (even that found in "healthy" whole wheat products)

• Refined corn

• Corn syrup and high-fructose corn syrup

While this list may seem short, these unhealthy carbs make up the majority of calories consumed in the modern diet. They are calorie-dense but nutrient-deplete, and quickly break down into glucose in the bloodstream, causing a rapid insulin spike. Refined wheat and corn might as well be pure sugar to your body since they are so quickly converted to glucose. While glucose is a form of energy our bodies are designed to use, we are simply not designed to handle the *quantity* of glucose the modern diet throws at us. The human body likes and operates well on a constant and steady stream of sugar into the blood. It does not like and does not operate well on heaping dumps of sugar, which it must work in overdrive to balance.

Sugar's scary cousin, high-fructose corn syrup, is one of the largest sources of calories in the modern diet right now. It's in everything from bacon to beer. High-fructose corn syrup is estimated to be twenty times more damaging in terms of the effect of high blood sugar than is regular old sugar. This is because it metabolizes faster than sugar, resulting in the nasty blood sugar spikes that undermine health and damage the skin.

Now, some diets call for very low to no carbohydrates so as to prevent the unhealthy blood sugar spike. But as we've discussed, not all carbohydrates are bad! In fact, healthy sources of carbohydrates are jam-packed with beauty-boosting minerals, vitamins, enzymes and fiber. Many of these micronutrients also carry antioxidant and anti-inflammatory properties and support the liver's natural detoxification pathways, further supporting skin health from within. As we discussed in the previous chapter, fresh fruits and vegetables should make up the majority of your carbohydrate intake, with a smaller amount coming from gluten-free grains and legumes.

Of course, these healthy sources of carbohydrates vary in their effect on blood sugar levels. The glycemic index is a tool that assigns a value to foods based on how quickly they increase blood glucose levels, and it is helpful when learning to manage blood sugar levels. But it only tells part of the story—it does not take serving size into account. This is why it's even more important to consider the glycemic load, another value that gives a more realistic picture of a food's impact on blood sugar levels. The slow release of glucose from low-glycemic foods helps to keep blood sugar levels steady. Most fresh fruits and vegetables have low glycemic loads, with the exception of white potatoes, sweet potatoes, ripe bananas, figs and grapes. Dried fruit and fruit juice (even fresh-squeezed) have an extremely high glycemic load and so should be limited in order to keep blood sugar levels steady.

EVER WONDER WHY YOU "REALLY NEED THAT COOKIE AND NEED IT NOW"?

Well, sugar truly is addicting. When you eat that cookie—or sugar in any other form—dopamine is released. Dopamine is a neurotransmitter that triggers feelings of reward and pleasure. It's released when we have sex, drink caffeinated beverages and/or partake in addictive drugs. It's called a "sugar high" for good reason. And as with drugs, the body craves more sugar after the high.

Even more significant: An extreme spike in blood sugar as is typical of a sugary or high-carbohydrate meal causes blood sugar levels to plummet below normal once they fall. When this happens, the body feels an emergency need to get it back up again ASAP. How can it best do so? With more sugar!

But don't worry—winning the battle against your sweet tooth becomes easier and easier. As your blood sugar levels balance, you will experience fewer sugar cravings since your body won't feel the extreme need to get blood sugar levels back up after crashing. In other words, you won't feel that "I need a cookie and I need it now!" urge that comes along with a sugar crash.

Using protein and fat to offset the natural sugars contained in healthy carbohydrates will ensure your skin gets all of the nutrients necessary for a naturally gorgeous glow without the radiance-robbing insulin spike.

Adjusting the macronutrient ratio of your diet is key to balancing blood sugar levels. Since protein and fat are digested more slowly, they slow the absorption of glucose into the bloodstream. This ensures your body gets the steady stream of sugar into the blood on which it thrives. Protein and fat also keep us feeling fuller longer. This is very important to overcoming those urges to drop everything and grab the nearest donut. Because if you are feeling full and satiated, you can much more easily say, "No, thank you, donut! You are terrible for my health and skin and I deserve better."

Again, the correct macronutrient ratio varies from person to person since we're all biologically unique. But getting 30 percent of your daily calories from protein, 30 percent from fat and 40 percent from healthy carbohydrates is a good starting place for keeping blood sugar levels steady. Consider these rough approximations rather than absolute, and adjust according to your needs.

Breakfast is the most important time of day to keep blood sugar levels balanced. Steady blood sugar levels at breakfast will continue on to lunchtime, preventing the cravings for sweets and energy slumps that are typical of the blood sugar roller coaster and have you grabbing for sugar. The ideal morning meal is packed with protein, includes a generous amount of healthy fat and contains some low-glycemic, complex carbohydrates. The Sweet Pepper Mini Frittatas (page 96) and Berry Satisfying Chia Pudding Parfait (page 99) are great breakfast options!

When seeking a little sweetness, a few natural sweeteners that contain skin-loving goodies can be used as healthier alternatives to sugar.

These natural, unprocessed sweeteners are high in natural sugars (hence their sweetness!) and so should not be consumed in excess, but are a superior alternative to refined sugar. If you have eliminated refined sugar and simple carbohydrates from your diet and have balanced your macronutrient ratios, there is nothing wrong with adding a bit of these sweeteners to your daily coffee or tea or using them to bake a sweet treat.

COCONUT SUGAR: Coconut sugar is one of my favorite healthy sweeteners. It tastes like brown sugar and contains beneficial minerals, such as the skin-loving zinc as well as the fiber inulin, which helps slow glucose absorption.

RAW HONEY: Raw honey contains antiaging antioxidants and enzymes.

PURE MAPLE SYRUP: Amazingly delicious, pure maple syrup contains decent amounts of glow-getting manganese and zinc. But be sure to take a close look at the ingredient label: Most of the syrups sold at the grocery store do not contain pure maple syrup but rather skin-sabotaging high-fructose corn syrup with maple flavoring.

BLACKSTRAP MOLASSES: Molasses is a thick syrup produced when the sugarcane plant is processed to make refined sugar. But unlike refined sugar, molasses carries some significant health benefits—it is rich in iron, potassium, vitamin B_6, magnesium, calcium and antioxidants. Be sure to select unsulfured, organic sugarcane molasses.

There is one more natural sweetener that appears to have very little to no effect on blood sugar levels.

STEVIA: The leaves from the stevia plant are amazingly sweet while not impacting blood sugar levels. When purchasing a stevia product, be sure to take a close look at the ingredient labels to avoid any sketchy additives. I prefer an organic liquid extract, of which I use just a few drops in a cup of tea.

Banana puree, dates, mashed sweet potato and applesauce are also often used in healthy baking recipes to provide natural sweetness.

Steady like a high school sweetheart. #BloodSugarGoals

Keeping your blood sugar levels in balance is one of the most important things you can do for the health of your skin. Not only are elevated blood sugar levels inherently damaging to the skin, but sugar and simple carbohydrates also trigger each of the other common culprits behind most skin issues. For this reason, you haven't heard the last about these troublemakers just yet!

SUPPORT YOUR GUT (YOUR SKIN WILL THANK YOU)

THE NOT-SO-GLAMOROUS GUTTY-WORKS HAVE MORE TO DO WITH BEAUTY THAN YOU'D THINK

"We want to stress once again the importance of a close collaboration between gastroenterologists and dermatologists, because the gastrointestinal system and the skin may be considered more and more 'two sides of the same coin.'"

–V. BONCIOLINI ET AL., "Cutaneous Manifestations of Non-Celiac Gluten Sensitivity: Clinical Histological and Immunopathological Features," *Nutrients* (2015).

Although not intuitive at first, the gut and the skin are very intimately connected.

Remember all of the glow-getting nutrients your skin is craving? Well, they're worth diddly-squat if digestion is impaired—if you're not properly breaking down those nutrients, your body simply can't make use of them. They go to waste (literally, many of the nutrients will be flushed down the toilet with your waste).

But the role of the gut extends far beyond simply breaking down foods and assimilating nutrients (though this is by no means simple). It's now known that up to 80 percent of the immune system resides in the gut and that the gut's microbiome is responsible for synthesizing a number of critical vitamins. And when there are imbalances and irritations in the gut, it is a significant source of chronic inflammation that often manifests elsewhere in the body, especially the skin.

The integrity of the gut lining plays a particularly significant role in skin health. Increased intestinal permeability, or "leaky gut," occurs when the delicate intestinal lining becomes permeable as a result of irritation to the gut lining. Inflammatory skin conditions, such as acne, eczema, dermatitis and rosacea, are actually considered one of the telltale signs of leaky gut by practitioners.

Needless to say, it's important that everything happening between your tongue and your tushie runs smoothly.

When it comes to supporting your gut for healthy skin, it's a matter of:

1. Eating for optimal digestion

2. Further supporting digestion when needed

3. Nourishing your gut microbiome

4. Protecting and healing your gut lining

Many of us simply aren't eating correctly, which impairs digestion and robs the skin of beautifying nutrients.

Yes, there is a wrong way to eat!

I know, this sounds a little silly. How could something so seemingly simple be done wrong? "Chewing my food? Psh, I've been doing that since I've had teeth!" But the digestive process is anything *but* simple and one that requires things go smoothly from beginning to end—when the process goes awry at the beginning, it can create a domino effect and impact other stages of the process further down the line (or really, further down the GI tract).

Luckily, this vital aspect of the digestive process is something you can remedy immediately. Even if you're midbite or the kitchen timer is going off, you can improve your digestion right now by breaking some bad habits and keeping a few rules in mind.

TAKE A DEEP BREATH AND RELAX

The digestive process begins even before any food touches your lips. Since it is a parasympathetic process ("rest and digest" mode), your body needs to be relaxed for it to run smoothly. When your body is stressed or in a sympathetic state ("fight or flight" mode), the body prioritizes the stress functions over the digestive functions. As a result, digestion is stalled and food is not properly broken down. This not only causes gas and bloating, but also prevents the skin from accessing vital, beautifying nutrients. Over time, this can lead to more serious issues, such as leaky gut, which triggers an inflammatory cascade that wreaks havoc for the skin.

Simply taking a deep relaxing breath or saying grace before beginning your meal can help you switch from sympathetic to parasympathetic mode. And if you're feeling stressed or on the run, it's best to wait until you are in a relaxed state before eating.

HOLD YOUR HORSES AND ACTUALLY CHEW YOUR FOOD

Chewing is an important digestive process in and of itself. When you eat too quickly, food will not be mechanically broken down enough, placing a burden on the stomach. Chewing also stimulates the secretion of saliva, which contains an enzyme that is essential for carbohydrate digestion, salivary amylase. Without this enzyme present, carbohydrates will not be properly digested and the sugars will ferment in your GI tract. This means gas, bloating and irritation to the intestinal lining.

Aim to chew each mouthful twenty to thirty times. If you find yourself speed-eating, try setting your utensils down after each bite and do not pick them up again until after you have swallowed. Slowing down will also help you be more in tune with how your body is feeling and prevent you from overeating, another bad habit that impairs digestion and we'll talk about more shortly!

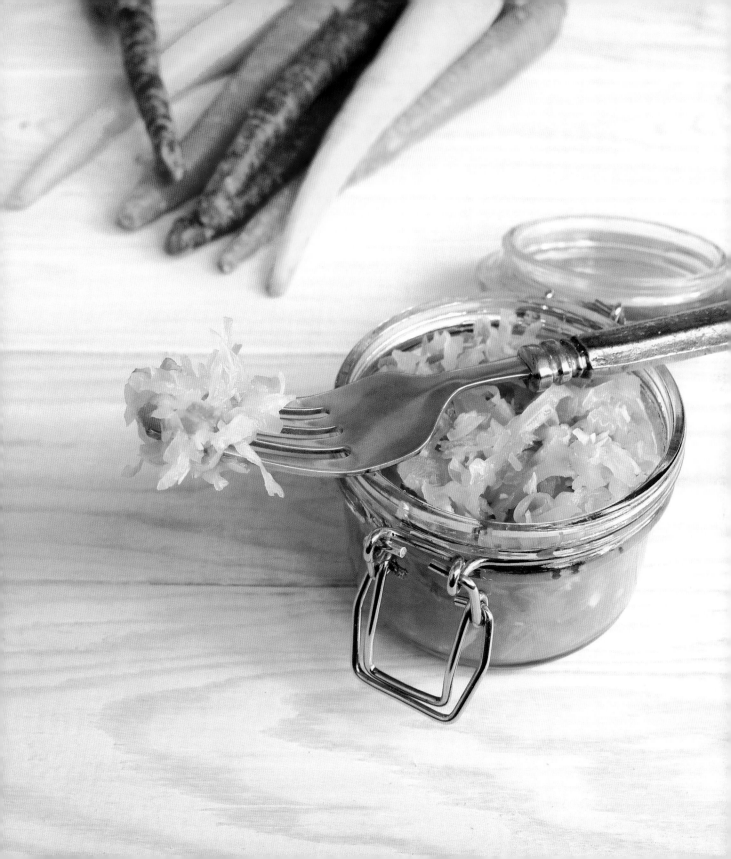

DON'T DRINK ANYTHING WHILE EATING

You may have heard that you should drink plenty of water with your meals to fill up your stomach and prevent you from overeating. This is absolutely terrible advice because doing so will impair digestion by diluting the gastric juices. This is especially important when eating protein, since proper hydrochloric acid levels are required to break down proteins into the amino acids necessary to build strong, healthy skin cells. And like undigested carbohydrates, undigested proteins can putrefy and irritate the gut lining.

It's best to stop drinking twenty minutes before eating and to avoid drinking for another twenty minutes after you have finished your meal. Of course, if you need to take supplements or medication with your meal, by all means drink! But try to limit it to a few sips to get the pills down.

STOP EATING WHEN YOU FEEL 80 PERCENT FULL

Have you ever noticed how uncomfortable you feel when you overeat? Well, it's more than just surpassing your stomach's carrying capacity—overeating stresses the entire digestive system. When the stomach's carrying capacity is exceeded and it can't fully digest your meal, that undigested load then continues on to the rest of the digestive organs, where it rancidifies and ferments. This causes gas and bloating, and irritates the intestinal lining.

Since it takes your stomach about twenty minutes to communicate with your brain, letting you know it's full, when you feel 80 percent full, you're very likely actually 100 percent full. So, putting the fork down when you feel 80 percent full prevents you from overeating.

This one is tough if you grew up in a household that rewarded you for finishing all of the food on your plate. Plus, chronically overeating can actually turn off the stomach's muscle memory that alerts the brain that you are full, making the habit even more difficult to break. However, you can reset this mechanism in about a week or so by strictly avoiding overeating during this time.

NOTE: If overeating is a problem for you, you'll find that balancing blood sugar levels also helps with this because your body never reaches the "crisis" point that accompanies a blood sugar crash.

Sometimes, the digestive system requires a bit more assistance.

If you're taking the steps to eat for optimal digestion but still experiencing symptoms of indigestion, such as bloating, burping or gas, you may need to further support digestion.

USE BITTERS OR APPLE CIDER VINEGAR TO STIMULATE GASTRIC JUICES

It's estimated that 50 to 90 percent of adults produce too little stomach acid. As soon as we see, smell, or think about food, our stomach cells begin secreting hydrochloric acid (HCl). HCl plays a vital role in protein digestion by converting pepsinogen into the enzyme pepsin, which breaks proteins down into amino acids. It also promotes the digestion and absorption of carbohydrates, fats and the glow-getting vitamins A and E by stimulating the release of pancreatic enzymes and bile into the small intestine. So, without adequate stomach acid, food is incompletely digested and nutrients are not properly assimilated. (And if you're thinking "Oh, well, I have acid reflux/gastroesophageal reflux disease [GERD], so I make too much stomach acid," think again. Contrary to popular belief, acid reflux and GERD are actually caused by low stomach acid. So, although antacids do help to alleviate the symptoms, they do not remedy the underlying cause.)

A few drops of bitters or 1 tablespoon (15 ml) of apple cider vinegar in a few ounces of water taken before a meal can help stimulate hydrochloric acid production.

EAT YOUR BEETS FOR BILE FLOW

Inadequate bile secretion is another common cause for indigestion. If we're not releasing enough bile to completely emulsify fats, our bodies can't absorb all of those beautiful-cell-building fatty acids and the fat-soluble, glow-getting vitamins A, D, E and K.

Especially if you've been eating a primarily low-fat diet, your body may need help digesting fat at first—when the gallbladder hasn't been called on to release bile in a while, it gets sluggish and the stored bile thickens. Beets are rich in betaine, which thins bile and aids fat digestion.

IF YOUR GALLBLADDER IS M.I.A., SUPPLEMENT WITH OX BILE

Although the liver is still producing bile, the gallbladder is not there to store and release it when you eat a fatty meal. So, instead, the bile slowly drips from the liver to the small intestine. Most often, there is an inadequate amount of bile present to digest a meal with even a moderate amount of fat.

Ox bile is just what it sounds like—bile from oxen—and is almost identical to our own bile. Taking an ox bile supplement when consuming fat will ensure it is being properly digested so your body and skin can reap all of the benefits.

The gut's microbiome needs special care and attention to keep skin healthy and glowing.

Our GI tract is home to trillions—around 100 trillion, in fact—of bacteria. The bacteria that make up our gut microbiome actually outnumber the cells in our bodies ten to one! Before you get grossed out and start thinking we're actually just walking, talking masses of bacteria, know that these bacteria are much smaller than our body cells, and collectively only weigh around 5 pounds (2.3 kg). Although they may be small, oh are these babies mighty—within recent years, more and more science has emerged confirming the connection between the gut microbiome and overall health, both physical and mental.

Like any good action movie (and the GI tract certainly is action-packed), the gut microbiome consists of good guys and bad guys. The good guys wear many hats: They aid digestion in the large intestine, manufacture the glow-getting vitamins B_7 (biotin), B_{12} and K_2 and produce short-chain fatty acids, which not only keep skin hydrated and supple but are also hard-hitters when it comes to fighting the inflammation that ages the skin prematurely and triggers acne and eczema. The bad guys, on the other hand, produce skin-damaging toxins and cause inflammation, which places an added burden on our bodies' natural detoxification processes and liver, which can further inflame the body and impact hormone balance. When all goes well, bad gut bacteria are kept in check by the healthy bacteria, but it is a delicate balance. So, we need to be sure that we're properly nourishing the good bacteria and keeping the bad bacteria under control.

EAT PLENTY OF PROBIOTIC-RICH FOODS

Try to get at least two servings of probiotic-rich foods—raw milk yogurt, raw milk kefir, water kefir, sauerkraut, kimchi, pickled veggies—into your diet daily. But commercial yogurt and kefir found in most grocery stores are to be avoided since they typically contain a lot of sugar and the bacterial cultures used are often very short-lived (so there may not even be any remaining probiotics in the product by the time you eat it).

FEED THE GOOD BACTERIA HIGH-QUALITY SOLUBLE FIBER AND RESISTANT STARCH

Soluble fiber acts as a prebiotic, a food for the good gut bacteria. Good sources of soluble fiber include chia seeds, flaxseeds, hemp fiber/protein, properly soaked and sprouted gluten-free grains, and fruits and vegetables (especially sweet potatoes and raw carrots with the skin on).

Resistant starch is a particularly fantastic prebiotic. It is called *resistant* since it resists digestion and absorption, passing right on to the large intestine where it becomes food for healthy gut bacteria. Good sources of resistant starch include green-tipped (not quite ripe) bananas, green plantains, white potatoes that have been cooked and then cooled to room temperature, white rice that has been cooked and then cooled to room temperature, cassava starch, potato starch and lentils.

STARVE THE BAD BACTERIA BY CUTTING OUT SUGAR AND SIMPLE CARBOHYDRATES

(Here they are again!)

Sugar and simple carbohydrates feed the "bad bacteria" and unhealthy yeasts in the digestive tract. This is yet another reason to eliminate all refined sugar and simple carbs from your diet. Individuals with a severely imbalanced microbiome may need to even avoid high-sugar fruits for a time as they work to bring things back into balance.

CHOOSE ORGANIC AS OFTEN AS POSSIBLE

Conventional fertilizers and pesticides can kill the good bacteria in the gut (and have a number of other toxic influences on your body).

It's also very important to take precaution when taking prescription antibiotics since they do not discriminate—they kill the good gut bacteria as well as whatever bad bacteria they were prescribed for! Only take prescription antibiotics when necessary (you don't typically need an antibiotic to get over a cold), and be sure to take a quality probiotic during and after the round of antibiotics, to repopulate the gut microbiome.

The integrity of the gut lining also greatly impacts the skin.

Increased intestinal permeability, or "leaky gut," occurs when the intestinal lining becomes permeable. To understand this concept and its implications, it helps to think of the gut lining as a screen door. The screen has teeny-tiny little openings that are big enough to allow fresh air to come into the house yet small enough to keep the buggies out. But what happens when your cat asserts his independence and pushes a hole into the screen? Your house is covered in creepy little outside invaders and you're not happy! You attack, swatting bugs left and right. Well, like a screen door, the gut lining is semipermeable. It is designed to allow nutrients that have been appropriately digested through to the bloodstream while keeping undigested foods out. But what happens when the integrity of the gut lining is compromised and there is a breach? Suddenly, undigested food particles enter the bloodstream. It's like having bugs in your house—the body sees these large, undigested food particles as outside invaders and is not happy! It attacks, signaling an immune response to fight these particles.

As mentioned at the beginning of the chapter, inflammatory skin conditions are considered one of the telltale signs of leaky gut. This is likely due to the fact that the immune response that results from leaky gut causes chronic inflammation. Leaky gut is also believed to be at the root of many food intolerances (not allergies), since the immune system holds a wicked grudge—it remembers its enemies so it can be better prepared to attack them in the future. So, if a specific type of undigested food leaks through your gut lining and triggers an immune response, it will likely happen again in the future so long as the lining is not repaired and that specific food continues to leak through. The presence of these undigested food particles and toxins in the blood also places an extra burden on the

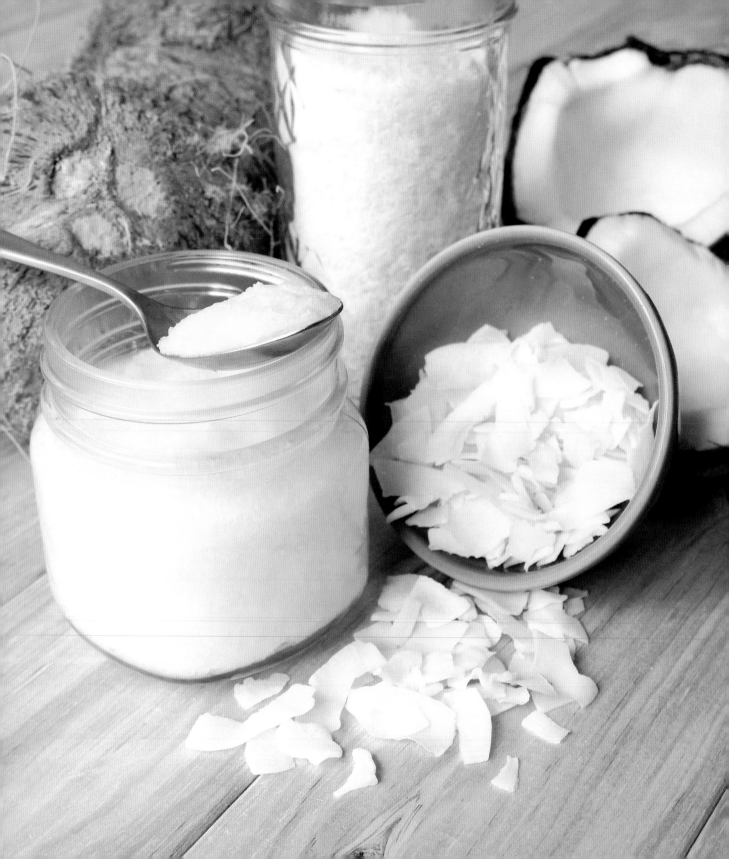

Improving digestion and nourishing the gut microbiome are key for keeping the gut lining healthy. Undigested foods can irritate the gut lining, promoting leaky gut. The short-chain fatty acids produced by the good gut bacteria not only keep skin glowing and reduce inflammation, but they also protect the gut lining. On the other hand, the bad gut bacteria create toxins that irritate the gut lining.

There are a few other impactful steps you can take to protect and repair your gut lining.

KICK GLUTEN TO THE CURB

Gluten has been shown to irritate the gut lining and trigger the release of zonulin, a chemical that signals the small spaces in the intestinal lining to open, allowing undigested food particles and toxins to enter the blood stream. This is a double whammy when it comes to increasing intestinal permeability.

SOAK GLUTEN-FREE GRAINS, LEGUMES, NUTS AND SEEDS TO INCREASE DIGESTIBILITY

These foods can be difficult to digest and so can easily irritate the gut lining. However, taking the extra step to soak grains, legumes, nuts and seeds before cooking or eating greatly increases their digestibility. Doing so also decreases their "antinutrient" content, which blocks mineral absorption in the gut.

Sprouting is the extra step beyond soaking. It further enhances digestibility and reduces antinutrient content as well as makes vitamins, enzymes, and minerals more bioavailable. This process is a bit more involved than soaking, but fortunately, many brands sell grains, legumes, nuts and seeds that have already been soaked and sprouted.

REPAIR YOUR GUT LINING WITH HEALING FOODS

Certain foods are all-stars when it comes to protecting and healing the gut lining. They include gelatin, bone broth (which is rich in gelatin), fermented vegetables, cabbage and coconut products. Your skin also loves these foods, so eat up!

Your skin will thank you for giving your gutty-works a little TLC.

By doing so, you'll be able to make the most of those glow-getting nutrients, ensure your immune system is operating at its best, adequately synthesize a number of vital glow-getting nutrients and reduce a primary cause of skin-irritating inflammation. Speaking of which . . . this leads us right into our next topic!

CALM SKIN-IRRITATING INFLAMMATION

A TOTAL GAME-CHANGER

Inflammation is a hallmark of such skin conditions as acne, eczema, dermatitis, premature aging and sun damage.

Yep, just about everything we want to avoid when it comes to our complexion!

So, it may be surprising to learn that inflammation is a necessary part of the body's natural healing response. When you get a cut on your finger, for example, the damaged cells produce chemical messengers that activate the inflammation process: Blood vessels dilate to increase blood flow to the area, white blood cells are released to attack foreign invaders like bacteria, and the finger swells to cushion and protect the damaged tissue. After this inflammatory and immune response is complete, anti-inflammatory chemicals move in to bring everything back to normal.

But acute inflammation and chronic (or systemic) inflammation are two totally different stories. A cut leads to acute inflammation that serves an immediate need and gets turned off when all is complete. An improper diet, on the other hand, consumed day after day and year after year, leads to chronic inflammation that never quite gets turned off. Chronic inflammation happens when the body sends an inflammatory response to a perceived internal threat that does not actually require an inflammatory response. The white blood cells are on alert but have no foreign invader to attack, and so sometimes eventually start attacking internal organs or other necessary tissues and cells. Chronic inflammation is at the basis of many diseases and chronic health conditions, from cancer to heart disease, Alzheimer's to arthritis. And as just mentioned, it's at the root of most skin issues as well.

Chronic inflammation is to blame for the classic signs of aging: wrinkles, loss of elasticity and sagging, discoloration and enlarged pores. In fact, the two are so intimately connected that they've earned themselves a celebrity couple nickname à la Brangelina (RIP): "inflammaging." Chronic inflammation is also a driving force behind such inflammatory skin conditions (whodathunk?) as acne, eczema, dermatitis and rosacea.

When it comes to calming skin-irritating inflammation, it's a matter of:

1. Adjusting your omega-6 and omega-3 essential fatty acid intake

2. Kicking pro-inflammatory ingredients and foods off your dinner plate

3. Adding some anti-inflammatory superstars to your diet

4. Neutralizing free radicals (both a cause and result of inflammation) with antioxidants

5. Identifying and eliminating food intolerances

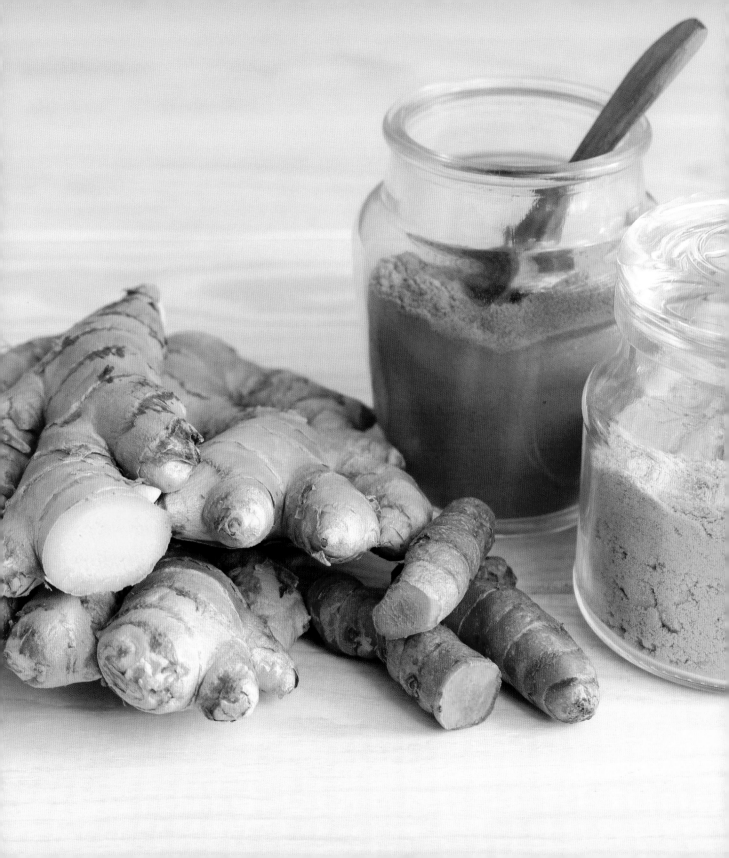

As we've already discussed, the modern diet does fat so, so wrong. It's loaded with omega-6 essential fatty acids and terribly lacking in omega-3 essential fatty acids. While both are indeed "essential" and regulate the inflammatory process, this imbalance promotes chronic inflammation. Omega-6 fatty acids are a necessary precursor to the chemical messengers that kick-start the inflammatory process. On the other hand, omega-3 fatty acids signal the chemical messengers that turn off the inflammatory process. Oily fish and marine algae are special sources of omega-3s since they contain EPA and DHA, which are converted into the anti-inflammatory compounds resolvins and protectins (yes, they sound like *resolve* and *protect*, which gives a hint as to what role they play in the body).

With the modern diet containing ten to fifteen times more omega-6 fatty acids than omega-3 fatty acids, our bodies are perfectly able to inflame without being able to adequately anti-inflame. This is a big problem. It's the perfect recipe for chronic inflammation.

Again, the body only requires a small amount of the essential fatty acids. So, don't worry about having to incorporate flaxseeds or salmon into each meal! The focus should be on reducing our excessive omega-6 fatty acid intake while increasing our omega-3 fatty acid intake.

OMEGA-3-RICH FOODS	OMEGA-6-RICH FOODS
Freshwater salmon	"Vegetable" oil
Sardines	Canola oil
Anchovies	Corn oil
Roe and caviar	Sunflower seed oil
Grass-fed beef	Safflower oil
Krill oil	Sesame oil
Chia seeds	Soybean oil
Flaxseeds*	Nuts and seeds

* Flaxseeds must be ground for your body to take advantage of their many health benefits. However, I do not recommend buying them preground since this accelerates the rate at which the delicate fatty acids go rancid. It's best to buy whole flaxseeds, store them in the refrigerator and grind them shortly before eating.

WHAT DOES THIS MEAN FOR SOME OF OUR FAVORITE NUTS AND SEEDS?

Nuts and seeds are inherently healthy, but it's important to know that they are a significant source of omega-6 fatty acids. Even walnuts, which are often touted as being a good source of omega-3s, have five times more omega-6s than 3s. So, I do suggest moderating your intake (i.e., don't go nuts with the nuts!), and balancing nuts and seeds rich in omega-6 fatty acids with healthy sources of omega-3 fatty acids.

A number of other common foods promote skin-irritating inflammation.

Removing these foods from your everyday diet will help to significantly reduce the systemic inflammation irritating the skin.

SUGAR + REFINED, SIMPLE CARBOHYDRATES

Ah, here they are yet again: our sweet skin saboteurs.

The insulin spike that accompanies an increase in blood sugar is extremely inflammatory. Elevated blood glucose levels can also damage proteins through the creation of AGEs, which trigger an inflammatory cascade in the body.

GLUTEN

As we discussed in the previous chapter, gluten damages the gut lining and can cause "leaky gut." By allowing toxins and undigested food particles to pass through the intestinal lining, leaky gut prompts an immune response and is a significant cause of chronic inflammation. A number of studies have confirmed this connection between gluten and inflammation and have found that gluten-free diets significantly reduced inflammatory markers.

OVERCOOKED FOODS

Pro-inflammatory AGEs aren't just a result of elevated blood sugar levels. They're also found in overcooked foods. It's best to avoid broiled, charbroiled, grilled, fried and burnt foods as often as possible. On the day-to-day, the best cooking options to minimize AGEs are boiling, steaming, slow-cooking, low-/medium-heat baking, and medium- to low-heat panfrying with a stable saturated fat.

FRIED FOODS

Not only are fried foods a source of dietary AGEs, they're also loaded with rancid "vegetable" oils. As we've discussed, not only are "vegetable" oils an unhealthy source of pro-inflammatory omega-6 essential fatty acids, but they should also never be heated. However, since they're very cheap oils, they're widely used in restaurants, including in the fry machine. When heated, the delicate polyunsaturated fats oxidize and become extremely pro-inflammatory.

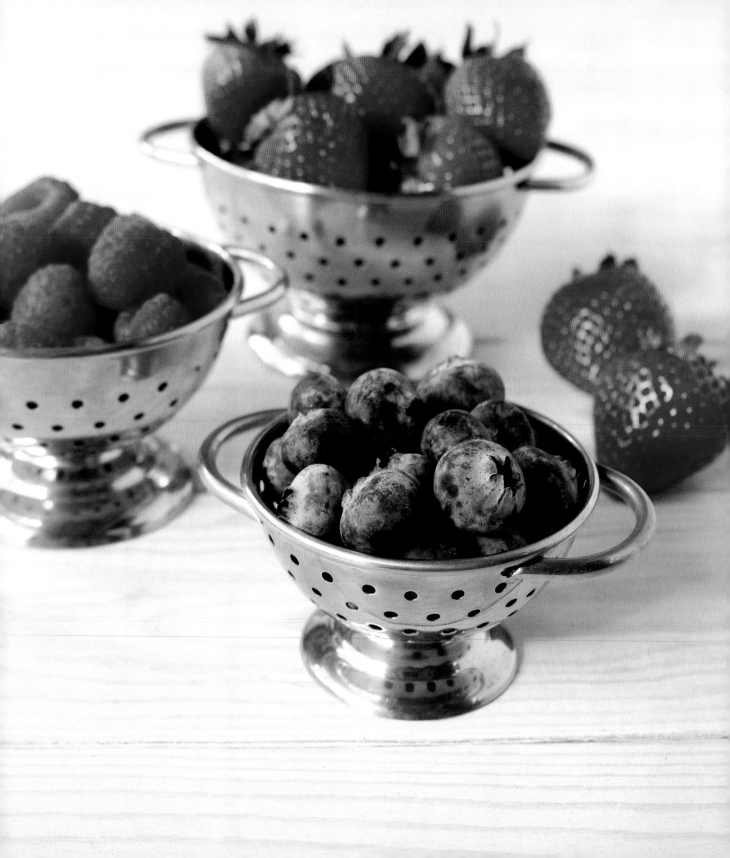

FRIED FOODS

Not only are fried foods a source of dietary AGEs, they're also loaded with rancid "vegetable" oils. As we've discussed, not only are "vegetable" oils an unhealthy source of pro-inflammatory omega-6 essential fatty acids, but they should also never be heated. However, since they're very cheap oils, they're widely used in restaurants, including in the fry machine. When heated, the delicate polyunsaturated fats oxidize and become extremely pro-inflammatory.

Some herbs and foods are anti-inflammatory superstars that your skin will love you for including in your diet.

These foods are as flavorful as they are powerful!

TURMERIC: The powers of this orange spice have not only been used in Ayurvedic medicine for centuries but have also been well studied. The curcumin contained in turmeric stops inflammation by blocking a molecule that switches on the genes related to inflammation.

GINGER: This spice has long been used in Ayurvedic medicine to reduce inflammation-related pain. Studies have shown that the flavonoid gingerol contained in ginger reduces pain in osteoarthritis patients as well as post-workout muscle soreness.

PINEAPPLE: The enzyme bromelain in pineapple is responsible for its anti-inflammatory effects. Research has shown that bromelain helps block the production of certain molecules that trigger inflammation.

ONIONS: Onions are rich in the flavonoid quercetin, which also helps reduce inflammation before it begins by blocking the synthesis of the messenger molecules that start the inflammatory process.

Check out the Tropical Turmeric Ice Pops (page 112) and Good Morning Anti-Inflammatory Elixir (page 116) for some ideas on how to incorporate these anti-inflammatory powerhouses into your diet.

Free radicals are both a result and cause of inflammation that need to be neutralized for glowing skin from within.

Free radicals are atoms or molecules with an unpaired electron in their outermost shell, rendering them unstable. They tear electrons away from other, stable molecules, creating a chain reaction. It's no wonder we most often hear about free radicals in light of antiaging: Free radicals destroy collagen. They can also damage cell membranes and DNA, causing cellular dysfunction, and oxidize the fats that make up the skin's sebum, which research suggests may increase the risk of blemishes. Just as threatening to the integrity of the skin, free radicals cause inflammation—though they last for only a fraction of a second, they initiate an inflammatory cascade that can go on for hours or days. This not only accelerates aging but can also exacerbate inflammatory skin issues.

The skin in particular is exposed to a great number of free radicals, thanks to environmental pollutants and as a result of sun exposure (which is why this topic will come up again when we discuss topical skincare). But as terrible as they seem, free radicals are a natural part of our system—they're by-products of the body's metabolism. In fact, every time we simply breathe, free radicals are created. Inflammation increases the rate at which these free radicals are created by the body, which yes, then go on to promote more inflammation! It's a vicious cycle that needs to be stopped.

WATERCRESS: Not only is watercress loaded with the antioxidant vitamins C and (preformed) vitamin A, but it's also rich in antioxidant flavonoids, which help protect against cellular damage and may also assist DNA repair. Interestingly, the "father of medicine," Hippocrates, is said to have established his first hospital near a watercress stream so he could use it to help treat his patients.

BLUEBERRIES: These little berries are well known for containing more antioxidants than most other fruits and vegetables. Equally important, they're also lower in sugar than are most other fruits, decreasing the risk of the pro-inflammatory insulin spike that accompanies an increase in blood sugar.

TOMATOES: Tomatoes are rich in the antioxidant lycopene, which has been proven to protect against the effects of UV radiation and reduce the risk of sunburn. Keep in mind that the lycopene is fat-soluble and four times more bioavailable (that is, it's more readily absorbed and assimilated by the body) in cooked tomatoes than raw tomatoes.

GREEN TEA: Green tea is loaded with catechins, a flavonoid and extremely potent antioxidant. Several studies have found that the catechins in green tea protect skin cells from oxidative stress and free radical damage. Vitamin C protects the catechins in green tea, making them up to five times more powerful once they're in your body. Yes, five times! So, be sure to squeeze some lemon in your iced green tea to get more bang for your antioxidant buck.

CACAO: Chocolate lovers, rejoice! Cacao is rich in flavonol, a type of flavonoid that has antioxidant and anti-inflammatory properties. Bonus: It also helps increase blood and oxygen circulation to the skin. But before you go grabbing for the nearest chocolate bar, remember to look for a high cacao content (I personally prefer over 75 percent) and to avoid unhealthy additives. Also keep in mind that unrefined cacao has a greater antioxidant content than processed cocoa (yes, the two sound and appear very similar but are actually different). Check out the AvoCacao Pot de Crème (page 103) to get your antioxidant and chocolate fix!

"EVERY BOY AND EVERY GIRL, SPICE UP YOUR LIFE!"

When making the transition to real food, some people feel that their meals are bland or they get stuck in a cooking rut, making the same meal over and over. Spices add amazing flavor to meals and are a great way to mix things up. But even more important, spices are a rich source of phytonutrients, most of which have potent antioxidant effects. Be sure to buy nonirradiated herbs and spices since the process of irradiation significantly reduces the phytonutrient content and natural medicinal properties. Certified organic spices are nonirradiated and the best choice.

Unidentified food intolerances are a significant source of systemic inflammation, accelerating skin aging and triggering pesky skin issues, such as acne and eczema.

You may not realize it, but the foods you eat every day may be causing systemic inflammation that's bankrupting your health and sabotaging your skin. With one in two individuals suffering from unidentified food intolerances, there's a 50 percent chance you are among them!

Now, there is a big difference between a food intolerance and a food allergy. Only 1 to 2 percent of the population suffers from a true food allergy. Food allergies are triggered by a particular protein within a food, to which the immune system responds with IgE antibodies. Food intolerances, on the other hand, can be triggered by any specific nutrient that incites an IgG antibody immune response. IgG antibodies react much more slowly than do their fast-acting IgE cousins, which is why symptoms of food intolerances can take up to a few days to present themselves. This delayed reaction makes identifying food intolerances tricky.

Signs of food intolerance range but often include:

- Persistent GI distress even with "clean eating" and digestive support
- Tiredness
- Brain fog
- Moodiness
- Joint stiffness or pain
- Headaches
- . . . and of course, inflammatory skin issues, such as acne, eczema and rosacea

NOTE: If your throat tightens, you get hives or you experience anaphylaxis immediately after eating certain foods, consult a doctor ASAP as you may have a true food allergy as opposed to a food intolerance.

Food intolerances wreak havoc on the whole body system—aggravating a number of inflammatory diseases from irritable bowel syndrome to arthritis—but especially the skin. This is because food intolerances cause chronic inflammation, provoking inflammatory skin conditions, such as acne and eczema. Food intolerances are also a source of stress for the body, triggering the release of collagen-damaging cortisol that can disrupt the delicate endocrine system. And by causing GI distress, food intolerances inhibit the digestion and absorption of the glow-getting nutrients necessary to build healthy skin cells.

It is therefore critical to remove from your diet foods to which you are intolerant . . . at least for a period of time. Whereas most food allergies last a lifetime, it is believed that leaky gut (refer back to page 55 if you need a refresher on the subject) is the cause of many food intolerances and that some intolerances can even be overcome by healing the gut. But, of course, this healing process can take a significant amount of time and requires the removal of all irritants, foods to which the body is intolerant being at the top of the list.

Although your doctor or health practitioner can run specific tests to pinpoint food intolerances, there are two simple tests that you can do at home to identify possible trigger foods—Coca's pulse test and the elimination diet. Both require keeping a close eye on your diet and your body's response to your diet.

NOTE: If you have any major medical conditions or are under a doctor's care, be sure to discuss the elimination diet with your doctor beforehand.

With both Coca's pulse test and the elimination diet, there are an absolute ton of foods you could test. Like, all of the foods you ever eat! So, I recommend starting with the most common trigger foods that are a part of your diet. Remember: You don't necessarily need to eat these foods every single day for them to be causing a reaction! Even if you eat these foods just once a week, it is a good idea to test them. While these are the most common trigger foods, some people experience food intolerances that seem to come out of left field. Oranges? Onions? Tomatoes? It's possible! While it may take some time to identify your particular trigger food(s), your skin will thank you for your thorough detective work with a glowing, even complexion.

COCA'S PULSE TEST

Coca's pulse test is a simple yet effective way to identify food intolerances. Since trigger foods cause a stress response, eating them will make your pulse rate increase. And so with this test, we're looking for an increased pulse rate as an indication of a possible intolerance.

It is important to test only one food at a time. You may wish to start with the common trigger foods: dairy products, wheat/gluten, eggs, corn, soy, legumes and grains. Testing whole foods will provide you with more precise information than testing prepared foods with multiple ingredients. (Note: If you are taking a medication that controls your heart rate, such as a calcium-channel blocker or a beta-blocker, this test will likely not be accurate.)

Here's how it works:

1. Sit down, take a deep breath and relax.

2. Establish your baseline pulse by counting your heartbeat for one full minute. Write this number down.

3. Put a bite-size amount of a food in your mouth. Chew the food or hold it on your tongue for a full minute, but do not swallow it—your taste buds need ample time to communicate with your immune system.

4. After chewing the food or holding it in your mouth for a minute, retake your pulse for another full minute with the food still in your mouth. Be sure to write down the food and your pulse after chewing the food. If your pulse has increased by six beats or more, this is considered a stressful reaction to a likely trigger food.

5. Spit the food out (do not swallow it).

6. If you did not experience a stress reaction, go ahead and test the next food by repeating steps 2 to 5. If you experienced a stress reaction, rinse out your mouth with some pure water, spit the water out and wait a few minutes before retesting your pulse to see if it has returned to its baseline. Only once your pulse has returned to its normal rate should you go on to test the next food.

Since Coca's pulse test is not 100 percent leakproof, I suggest doing a modified elimination diet with the foods that caused an increased pulse rate to confirm whether you have an intolerance.

ELIMINATION DIET

The elimination diet works by removing a number of common trigger foods from your diet for three to four weeks, then testing them by reintroducing them back into your diet one by one. In essence, it gets you feeling great so you can then easily identify those foods that make you feel not so great. More than simply a tool to identify food intolerances, the elimination diet is a great way to press the reset button on your diet and reduce skin-aggravating systemic inflammation.

That being said, doing the elimination diet properly takes dedication and discipline. And really, there's no reason to do it at all if you're not going to do it properly, since the IgG antibodies released in response to a food intolerance can take up to three weeks to work their way out of your system. So, if you're strict with the diet for seven days, then have a "cheat day," that single day of decadence may undo all of your hard work in the first week and you'll need to start from square one!

Although it may seem impossible to be so strict with your diet for such an extended period of time, it will be worth it. In and of itself, being able to easily identify and so avoid your trigger food(s) is an extremely satisfying, empowering feeling. This gives you such important insight into your unique body and health. Just as important, many people experience increased energy, better sleep, reduced pain and better mental health after successfully doing the elimination diet. Oh, and one more to add to this list: radically improved, glowing skin.

Of course, your body may experience an adjustment period before reaping these rewards. "Healing reactions" are quite common and can include headaches, lightheadedness, disrupted sleep and even GI issues—yes, all the opposite of all of those lovely benefits I just told you about! If these reactions are severe, be sure to seek medical attention. But if they are mild, continue on with the diet and keep in mind that they are simply symptoms of your body returning to balance.

Here's how it works:

1. Pick a five- to six-week period during which when you can realistically commit to properly doing the elimination diet—three to four weeks for the elimination period, and two to three weeks (though you may possibly need more time here) for the reintroduction period. Around the holidays or during a family vacation would not be a great time to do so, since there are likely to be so many temptations surrounding you and slim pickings at parties and restaurants!

2. Make note of your particular skin issues as well as other possible symptoms of food intolerances, such as digestive issues, joint pain, allergies, brain fog, low energy and mood issues. You will be keeping a close eye on how these symptoms progress during the elimination diet and the reintroduction period.

3. In the days before you begin your diet, stock your refrigerator and pantry with all of those foods to include in the diet. If you think you may give into cravings too easily, get the foods that need to be eliminated out of your house! And remember to look closely at the ingredient labels of packaged foods to ensure they do not contain any of the foods to eliminate.

	FOODS TO INCLUDE	FOODS TO ELIMINATE
FRUITS	All except citrus fruits	Citrus fruits
VEGETABLES	All except corn and nightshades	Corn and nightshade vegetables (potatoes, tomatoes, eggplant, peppers)
GRAINS	Brown rice, millet, quinoa, amaranth	Wheat, corn, barley, spelt, Kamut, rye, oats

	FOODS TO INCLUDE (CONTINUED)	FOODS TO ELIMINATE (CONTINUED)
LEGUMES	-----	All legumes (including soy and soy products)
NUTS AND SEEDS	-----	All nuts and seeds
MEAT, FISH AND EGGS	Fish, chicken, turkey, lamb, wild game	Eggs, beef, pork, cold cuts, bacon, hotdogs, canned meat, sausage, shellfish
DAIRY PRODUCTS AND NONDAIRY MILK SUBSTITUTES	Unsweetened nondairy milk substitutes	All dairy products
FATS	Extra-virgin olive oil, coconut oil, avocado oil	Butter, vegetable oil, canola oil, hydrogenated oil
BEVERAGES	Fresh water, herbal teas	Alcohol, coffee, caffeinated teas, soda
SPICES, CONDIMENTS AND FLAVORINGS	Sea salt, black pepper, fresh herbs and spices, raw cacao	Ketchup, mustard, relish, chutney, soy sauce, vinegar, BBQ sauce, chocolate
SWEETENERS	Stevia, coconut sugar	White and brown sugar, honey, maple syrup

During and after the diet:

1. For the three to four weeks you have set aside for the elimination period, indulge in the foods to include in the diet while abstaining from the foods to eliminate. Remember that this is not about calories! It is simply about giving your system a break and starting with a clean slate with which you can test for possible food intolerances.

(continued)

2. During the elimination period, make note of changes in your skin and other symptoms noted in step 2 of your preparation for the diet. The assumption and hope would be that they improve. Are they?

3. After the elimination period is complete, begin the reintroduction period. Start with the common trigger foods: wheat/gluten, dairy, eggs, soy, corn, peanuts, nightshades. Reintroduce just one food at a time: Eat the food on an empty stomach, and then carefully see how your body reacts over the next two days (during this time, you will have otherwise resumed the elimination diet). If your skin issues flare or the other symptoms noted in step 2 rear their ugly heads again, you know that you likely have intolerance to this food and that it should be cut from your diet. If there are no negative reactions, you can include the food back into your diet and move on to reintroducing another food.

Since the elimination diet is a common tool used by nutrition professionals and functional medicine practitioners, there are a ton of recipes and other useful resources online to help you as you work through the diet.

It's time to get a grip on runaway inflammation!

Simply adjusting your essential fatty acid intake, eliminating pro-inflammatory foods and adding anti-inflammatory and antioxidant-rich foods will dramatically decrease the inflammatory load on your body. And if you have a persistent inflammatory skin condition and/or the other symptoms of a food intolerance, taking the time to figure out if you intolerant to specific foods will be one of the best things you can do for your health and skin.

KEEP HORMONES HEALTHY AND SKIN HAPPY

BALANCE IS THE KEY

Hormones are chemical messengers that tell your body what to do, when to do it and how. Yeah, they're a pretty big deal.

There are dozens of different hormones in the human body, each with a vital function. The sex hormones androgens and estrogens and the stress hormone cortisol wield the most influence over the skin.

Any pubescent teen knows the intimate connection between the sex hormones and the skin, particularly acne. We typically start experiencing breakouts during adolescence, when androgen levels spike. This stimulates the sebaceous glands to grow and produce more sebum. Elevated androgen levels also increase the rate at which skin cells shed. When these shed skin cells get stuck in the pore, they trap the sebum and create a feasting ground for *P. acnes*. Yes, it is a perfect recipe for acne. But the connection between hormones and acne doesn't end when the clock strikes midnight on our twentieth birthday. Many adult women experience breakouts around menstruation and while pregnant—androgen levels increase before ovulation and in the first two trimesters of pregnancy, activating the sebaceous glands and increasing the opportunity for breakouts. For this reason, acne also typically accompanies polycystic ovary syndrome (PCOS), a female hormonal disorder that is characterized by elevated levels of androgens.

The stress hormone cortisol also greatly impacts the skin. Ever noticed how you may break out in blemishes or your eczema may flare when you are stressed? Well, cortisol creates an inflammatory state and stimulates the oil glands, increasing sebum production. Cortisol also reduces the skin's ability to retain moisture and is a supervillain when it comes to skin aging—it damages collagen and slows its rate of repair, inhibits the skin's synthesis of skin-plumping hyaluronic acid and thins the top layers of the skin. Chronic stress and high cortisol levels also impact the skin by throwing the sex hormones off balance—since the body prioritizes survival over reproduction, the adrenal glands use up all of the precursor hormone pregnenalone (aptly named pregnenalone steal), which is used to create both cortisol and the sex hormones.

When it comes to keeping hormones happy and skin healthy, it's a matter of:

1. Ditching the foods that raise acne-causing androgen levels

2. Removing stressors to put cortisol back in its place

3. Supporting the liver for proper hormone detoxification

Two particular foods have been shown to greatly exacerbate hormonal acne.

Hormonal acne is often cystic and is most prominent along the jawline, on the chin and around the mouth as well as on the back, thighs and bottom. If you experience this pattern of breakouts along with other telltale signs of hormonal imbalance—irregular periods, painful menstruation, worsening breakouts around menstruation, low libido—it is best to avoid these two foods.

SUGAR + REFINED, SIMPLE CARBOHYDRATES

We're now well aware that eating sugar and refined, simple carbohydrates causes a spike in blood sugar levels which causes a spike in insulin levels and causes inflammation, and that inflammation promotes everything we don't want to happen to our skin. But insulin also stimulates sebum production and increases the skin's sensitivity to androgen hormones, increasing the risk of acne.

DAIRY PRODUCTS

Dairy also stimulates the release of insulin and insulin-like growth factor 1. Both of these hormones stimulate sebum production and skin cell growth, stimulate androgen production and increase the skin's sensitivity to androgens. This is a triple whammy when it comes to increasing the risk of acne.

Dairy products also inherently contain hormones that can throw our own hormones off balance. Conventional dairy produced in factory farms is especially concerning since these operations typically inject cows with synthetic hormones to increase milk production.

If hormones are the primary cause of your acne, it's still very important to get the proper nutrients via a real food diet, support your gut and calm skin-irritating inflammation in addition to cutting these two problem foods so as to heal the skin from all angles.

It's critical for all of us to take particular steps to lower damaging cortisol levels.

Not only will this benefit the skin, but it will also make you generally healthier and happier since stress is a primary cause of chronic inflammation and just no fun either!

STRESS LESS

Okay, easier said than done, right? But look for small ways to reduce your stress throughout the day in whatever way you can, whether it's taking a five-minute walk outside during lunch, journaling, repeating positive affirmations or doing some deep-breathing exercises.

MAKE TIME FOR REST

This not only means getting a good night's sleep, but also not pushing your body too far with vigorous exercise. Eating after exercise helps to temper the stressful effect on the body and give it the nutrients it needs to build and repair.

IDENTIFY AND REMOVE FOOD INTOLERANCES

As we've discussed, food intolerances can be extremely taxing on the body and elevate cortisol levels. Some have likened the stress felt by the body from food intolerances to the stress felt from a stressful marriage or job. Refer back to pages 65–70 to learn how you can identify possible food intolerances.

EAT AN APPROPRIATE AMOUNT

Both undereating and binge-eating stress the body, increasing cortisol output. A very low-carbohydrate diet has also been shown to increase cortisol levels.

LIMIT CAFFEINE INTAKE

Another one that may be easier said than done! Drinking caffeinated beverages thrusts your body into a state of stress, even though you may feel perked up and ready to take on the day. It may especially be helpful to reduce caffeine if you experience other stressors that are not as easily controllable (such as a stressful job you are unable to leave).

The liver plays a tremendous role in hormone balance and deserves some extra TLC.

The liver is one hardworking organ—it's responsible for over 500 functions that are absolutely vital for our health, the most well known of which is detoxification. The liver filters a whopping 6 cups (1.4 L) of blood per minute, removing toxins. These toxins include excess and used hormones, as well as "dirty hormones" that mimic and interfere with our bodies' natural hormones.

While the liver was designed to handle its numerous tasks, there are a few aspects of modern life this organ was just not prepared for. We live in an increasingly toxic world: There are over 80,000 man-made chemicals used in industry today, most of which have never been tested for safety. We're not only exposed to these pollutants from air and water, but also from seemingly innocent everyday products, such as dish detergent, bed mattresses, carpeting and body wash. Once these chemicals enter the body, they're considered our "body burden." The liver is tasked with filtering, neutralizing and eliminating these toxins—on top of all its other responsibilities.

Our bodies are constantly bombarded by unhealthy chemicals, many of which interfere with the hormones. Many of these chemicals are considered "dirty hormones," "xenoestrogens" or "endocrine disruptors." They mimic our natural hormones and by doing so interfere with our endocrine system. The plasticizer BPA is a very well-known endocrine disruptor and one that we come into contact with very often.

The modern, nutrient-deplete diet also makes things extremely difficult for the liver. Imagine if the company you work for fired the two other members of your team and slashed your budget in half, but expected you to continue producing the same quality of work and meeting the same deadlines as before. Impossible, right? Although you'd be working overtime, your work would inevitably suffer. Well, this is what modern living and the modern diet are doing to the liver: They're increasing its workload (environmental toxins and unhealthy food ingredients that need to be detoxified) while reducing its resources (the vital nutrients it needs for the process of detoxification).

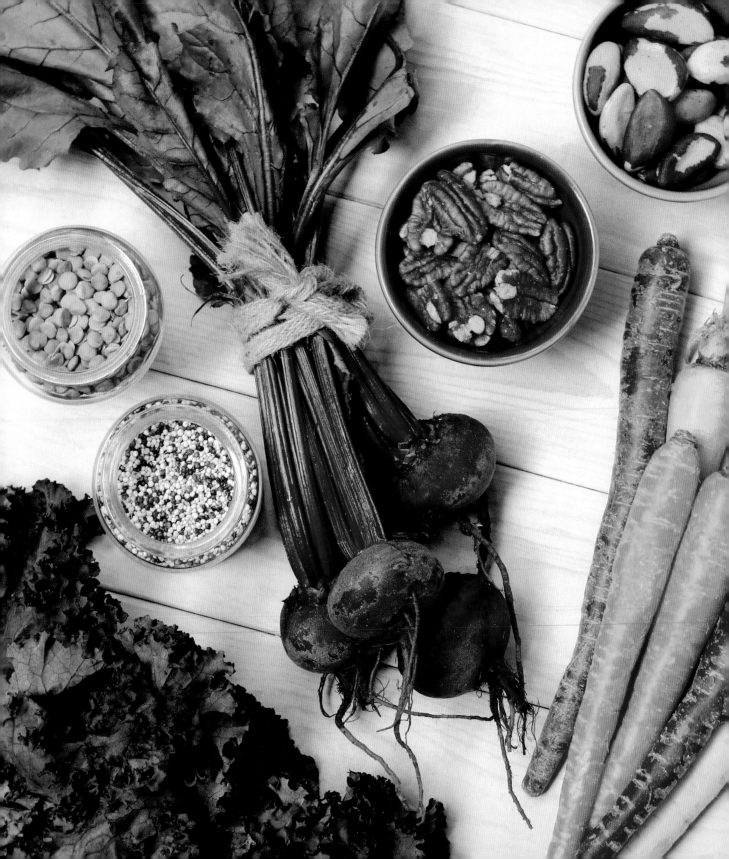

If the liver is not able to detox excess and used hormones as quickly as it needs to, they are reabsorbed into the body and put back in circulation. This causes hormonal excess. And since the endocrine system is very delicate, when one hormone is thrown off balance it can have a cascade effect on the other hormones.

By supporting the liver, we can help ensure excess and used hormones as well as "dirty hormones" entering our bodies from foods and the environment are properly and completely eliminated.

EAT A NUTRIENT-DENSE, REAL FOOD DIET

Of course!

The liver's phase 1 detoxification pathway (which essentially takes toxins and breaks them down) is dependent on the B vitamins, vitamins A, C, D and E, calcium, glutathione and carotenoids. A diverse, real food diet will help ensure that your liver has adequate amounts of these nutrients.

KEEP BLOOD SUGAR STEADY

The liver is a critical organ for blood sugar regulation—it stores or releases glucose based on the body's needs. Well, when blood sugar levels are erratic, the liver is constantly on call, working overtime to try and keep things steady. This is yet another reason that it's so important to keep blood sugar levels balanced!

INCLUDE PROTEIN AND FAT IN YOUR DIET

Hopefully, you're already including enough of these glow-getting macronutrients in your diet. If not, here's one more reason to do so: Amino acids from proteins are necessary for the liver's phase 2 detoxification pathway (in which the liver combines toxins with specific nutrients to make them less harmful and easier to excrete from the body—pretty darn important), and healthy fats are needed to create healthy, flowing bile to prevent stagnation.

INCREASE FIBER INTAKE

Bowel movements are one of the body's main detoxification routes—the liver eliminates toxins via bile, which is released into the small intestine to emulsify and absorb fat. Since fiber keeps us regular, it prevents the absorption of these chemicals back into the body (as can happen with constipation). Fiber also binds to these detoxed hormones, preventing them from being reabsorbed even if transit time is slower.

As with most nutrients, the average American eats far less fiber than she or he should: only around 15 grams of fiber per day. This is about half the suggested intake for women and a third of the suggested intake for men. To boost fiber intake, eat plenty of fresh fruits and vegetables with the skin on, as well as nuts, seeds and gluten-free whole grains. While increasing your fiber intake, do so gradually—adding fiber too quickly can upset your stomach. Try adding 5 grams each week until you reach your optimal level.

EAT YOUR BEETS FOR BILE FLOW

As mentioned on page 53, beets are rich in betaine, which helps thin viscous, stagnant bile. For this reason, beets not only help to digest fats but also move toxins from the body. Betaine is also a necessary cofactor for methylation, a key aspect of phase 2 liver detoxification pathway. The tops and greens of beets are actually the most potent (even more than the beets themselves), so don't throw them away! And if you've never been a big fan of beets, be sure to check out the Beet and Berry smoothie (page 115) for a delicious way to sneak them into your diet.

INCLUDE SOME LIVER-LOVING HERBS

Two herbs are powerhouses when it comes to protecting the liver: dandelion root (yes, the weed with the little yellow flower that grows in your backyard!) and milk thistle. Dandelion root stimulates bile flow and is rich in protective antioxidants. Milk thistle contains silymarin and silybin, antioxidants that protect the liver from toxins. Silymarin may also help to regenerate liver cells and helps boost levels of glutathione, a super-antioxidant that is crucial for liver detoxification.

> The endocrine system is extremely complex and certainly has no "overnight fix."

However, these small dietary tweaks can certainly help to bring things closer into balance, especially for the sake of the skin.

If you have ongoing signs of hormonal imbalance, I suggest seeking out the care of a functional medicine doctor who can help you pinpoint potential causes of the imbalance and work with you to restore proper hormonal levels holistically.

GLOW TIME

PUTTING IT ALL INTO PRACTICE

We just went over a TON of information about nutrition, our bodies and our skin.

If your head is spinning, don't worry! It will straighten itself out as you begin putting what you've learned into practice.

Again, everything you just read was in a specific order for a reason. For many people, simply cutting out processed foods and making the switch to a real food diet rich in glow-getting nutrients will be the key to supporting their skin from the inside out. They will find that inflammation is reduced, digestive issues disappear, hormones are healthy and in balance, and skin is glowing!

For others, things may not be quite so simple. But perhaps as you were reading you had a lightbulb moment and realized that a specific issue, such as impaired gut health or hormonal imbalance, has been nagging at you and needs to be addressed. If not, simply make your way through the sections one at a time.

Here's a quick recap of everything we've learned so far, to help you put it all into practice:

FEED YOUR SKIN THE NUTRIENTS IT'S CRAVING

- Make the switch to a real food diet.
  - Eat real food (duh).
  - Eat a variety of different real foods for an array of nutrients.
  - Eat real foods of all different colors to further ensure you're getting a broad spectrum of nutrients.
- Incorporate each of the glow-getting macronutrients in each meal.
  - Proteins are required to build and repair skin cells, which shed and regenerate constantly.
  - Carbohydrates provide cells with energy.
  - Fats are a necessary component of cell membranes. Healthy cell membranes make healthy cells, and healthy cells make healthy skin!
- Seek out the glow-getting micronutrients.
  - Not so difficult to do when you're incorporating the glow-getting sources of macronutrients in each meal!

GET OFF THE BLOOD SUGAR ROLLER COASTER

- Eliminate sugar, high-fructose corn syrup and refined, simple carbohydrates (wheat and corn) from the diet.

- Balance carbohydrates with adequate protein and fat. Although the "right" macronutrient ratio varies from person to person, getting 30 percent of your daily calories from protein, 30 percent from fat and 40 percent from healthy carbohydrates is a good starting place for keeping blood sugar levels steady. Consider these rough approximations rather than absolute, and adjust according to your needs.

- Use moderate amounts of natural, unprocessed sweeteners for a little extra sweetness. These include coconut sugar, raw honey, pure maple syrup and blackstrap molasses as well as stevia extract (which has little to no effect on blood sugar levels).

SUPPORT YOUR GUT

- Eat for optimal digestion by relaxing before beginning your meal, properly chewing your food, refraining from drinking while eating and stopping when you feel 80 percent full.

- When needed, further support digestion with bitters, apple cider vinegar, beets and ox bile supplementation.

- Nourish your gut microbiome by eating plenty of probiotic-rich foods and soluble fiber, and cutting out sugar and refined carbohydrates.

- Protect and heal your gut lining by removing gluten, soaking grains, legumes, nuts and seeds to enhance digestibility, and adding healing bone broth, gelatin, fermented vegetables, cabbage and/or coconut products to your diet.

CALM SKIN-IRRITATING INFLAMMATION

- Reduce omega-6 and increase omega-3 essential fatty acid intake.

- Kick pro-inflammatory ingredients and foods off your dinner plate. These include sugar, refined carbohydrates, gluten, overcooked food and fried food.

- Add some anti-inflammatory superstars, such as turmeric, ginger, pineapple and onions, to the menu.

- Neutralize free radicals with antioxidants. Particularly powerful sources include watercress, blueberries, tomatoes, green tea and cacao.

- Identify and eliminate food intolerances using the Coca's pulse test or elimination diet.

KEEP YOUR HORMONES HAPPY

- If you are experiencing hormonal acne, ditch dairy and sugar, which raise acne-causing androgen levels.

- Remove physical and emotional stressors to put cortisol back in its place. Make time for rest, eliminate foods to which you are intolerant from your diet, eat an appropriate amount and limit caffeine intake.

- Support the liver for proper hormone detoxification by increasing fiber intake and including some liver-supporting herbs and beets to your diet.

START SMALL AND THOUGHTFULLY

Maybe for you this means cutting out soda, sneaking some greens in with a daily smoothie or ditching sugar. Whatever it is, just start. You will find that once you do, the other changes come a lot more easily if not effortlessly.

And as you're working through the sections and putting it all into practice, keep in mind that you're making a tremendous investment—an investment in better health, one of the many rewards of which is glowing skin from within.

DON'T WORRY ABOUT THAT MYTHICAL THING CALLED "PERFECTION"

There are times when it's important to be very strict with your diet, such as if you have a food allergy or have been diagnosed with candida overgrowth and need to avoid carbohydrates for a period of time. But a healthy diet and lifestyle is all about balance, and (gasp!) this even includes occasional "cheats" and treats. So don't stress if you happen to step outside of the recommendations outlined in these pages or any other health plan!

Negative feelings like guilt and shame shouldn't surround food. In fact, the stress they incite is probably unhealthier than whatever it is you ate that's making you feel so negatively. It's important to accept that there is no such thing as "perfect" and to simply do the best you can.

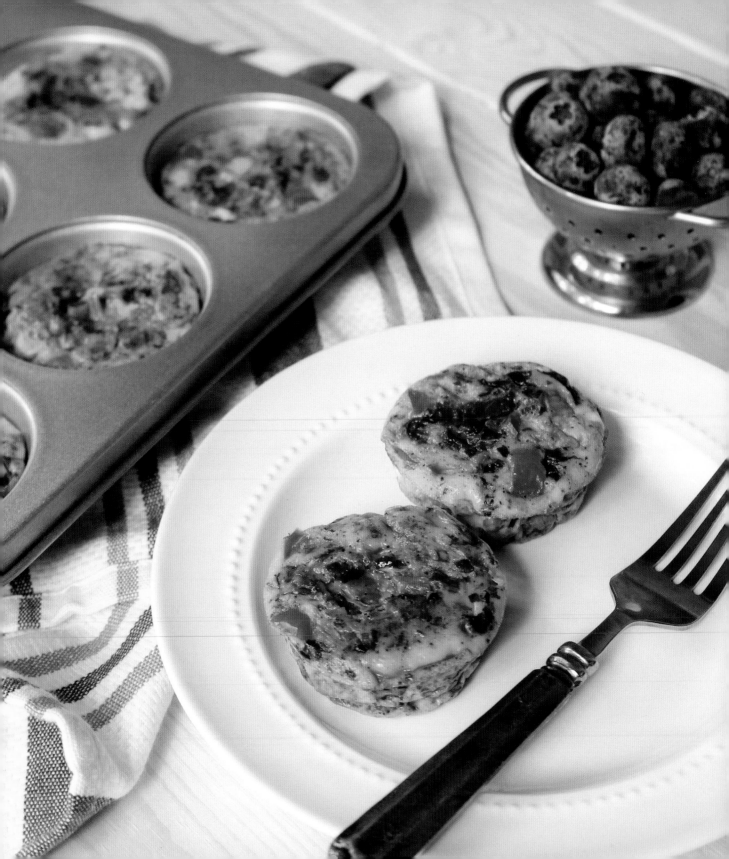

Skin-Loving Superfood Recipes

• • •

READY TO EAT YOUR WAY TO NATURALLY GORGEOUS SKIN?

IF ONLY DELICIOUS FOOD WAS THE ANSWER TO ALL OF LIFE'S TROUBLES!

These recipes all include healthy, whole, real food ingredients jam-packed with glow-getting nutrients.

They contain healthy fats and protein to not only build beautiful skin cells but also prevent the inflammatory insulin spike that accompanies a rise in blood sugar levels. You'll also find a few dishes where the anti-inflammatory powerhouse omega-3 fatty acid is the main event, and another that is as much about feeding your gut microbiome as it is about feeding you.

Each is free of the ultimate radiance-robbers—sugar and refined, simple carbohydrates—as well as gluten and dairy, since we now know that these are very common triggers for pesky skin issues.

It's important to make these recipes work for you!

If you have a nightshade or grain intolerance, for example, a few of these recipes will need to be tweaked or skipped.

But have fun and enjoy the process! Remember that food is a pleasure that has the power to make us feel really good . . . and look darn good, too.

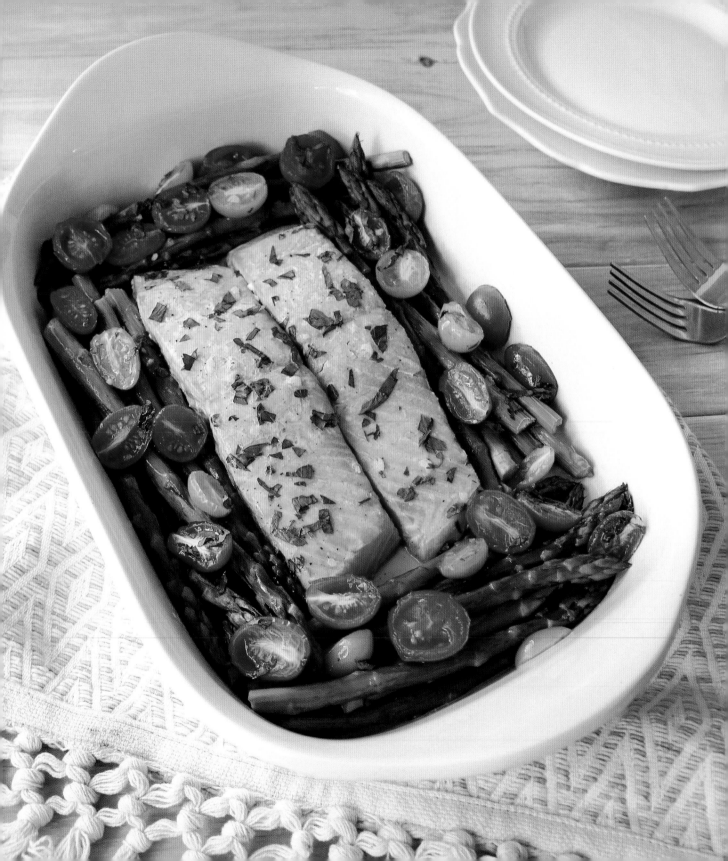

Single Sheet Baked Salmon and Veggies

If you're not in on the secret yet, here it is: Salmon is incredibly easy to cook up to gourmet perfection in no time flat. And with this particular dish, the salmon and side veggies are baked together at once. So, not only does it give your skin the glow-getting nutrients it craves and your taste buds quite a delight, but it also gives your life some of its precious time back. Wins all around!

Salmon is one of the best sources of anti-inflammatory omega-3 fatty acids, which we learned, back on page 60, are absolutely critical to fighting the inflammation that causes premature skin aging and fuels the fire behind inflammatory skin issues. Tomatoes protect skin with the antioxidant lycopene and an array of glow-getting vitamins. Asparagus provides cleansing fiber to help keep hormones in balance as well as provide protective antioxidants and vitamins.

YIELD: 2 SERVINGS

1 tsp (5 ml) avocado oil

1 bunch (350 g) asparagus

15 grape tomatoes

2 (6-oz [170-g]) wild salmon fillets

3 tbsp (11 g) fresh parsley, chopped

3 tbsp (45 ml) avocado oil

¼ cup (60 ml) freshly squeezed lemon juice

½ tsp mineral-rich sea salt

¼ tsp freshly ground black pepper

2 cloves garlic, peeled and minced

Preheat the oven to 350°F (180°C). Lightly grease a sheet pan or tempered glass baking dish with the avocado oil.

Remove the woody ends of the asparagus and cut the grape tomatoes in half.

Place the salmon fillets (skin side down) in the middle of the prepared pan and surround them with the asparagus and tomatoes.

Sprinkle the parsley over the salmon, asparagus and tomatoes.

In a small bowl, whisk the avocado oil, lemon juice, salt, pepper and garlic together, and drizzle over everything.

Bake for 22 to 26 minutes, or until the salmon is cooked to your liking.

NOTE: If you want to double this recipe, you'll need to use at least a 4-quart (3.8-L) baking dish or a half sheet pan.

Curried Avocado Chicken Salad

This twist on classic chicken salad has a little something to delight all your taste buds. It's sweet, savory and very satisfying. Best yet, it's jam-packed with glow-getting nutrients.

Avocado, chicken and pecans provide the skin with cell-building protein and fat, which also keep us feeling full and prevent an inflammatory insulin spike. Avocados are also loaded with cleansing fiber to aid the body's natural detox process and free radical–fighting antioxidants. The spices, grapes and celery not only add amazing flavor, but they also bring potent antioxidant power.

YIELD: 3 TO 4 SERVINGS

1 avocado

2 tsp (8 g) curry powder

⅛ tsp sea salt

1 lb (454 g) pasture-raised chicken, cooked and shredded or cubed

10 grapes, quartered

¼ cup (32 g) pecans, crushed

1 rib celery, diced

2 tbsp (8 g) chopped fresh parsley

In a mixing bowl, mash the avocado.

Add the curry powder and salt to the avocado, and stir to combine.

Add the chicken, grapes, pecans, celery and parsley to the avocado mixture, and stir everything together until you have a consistent mixture.

Serve alone, on a bed of greens, in lettuce wraps or on top of cucumber slices.

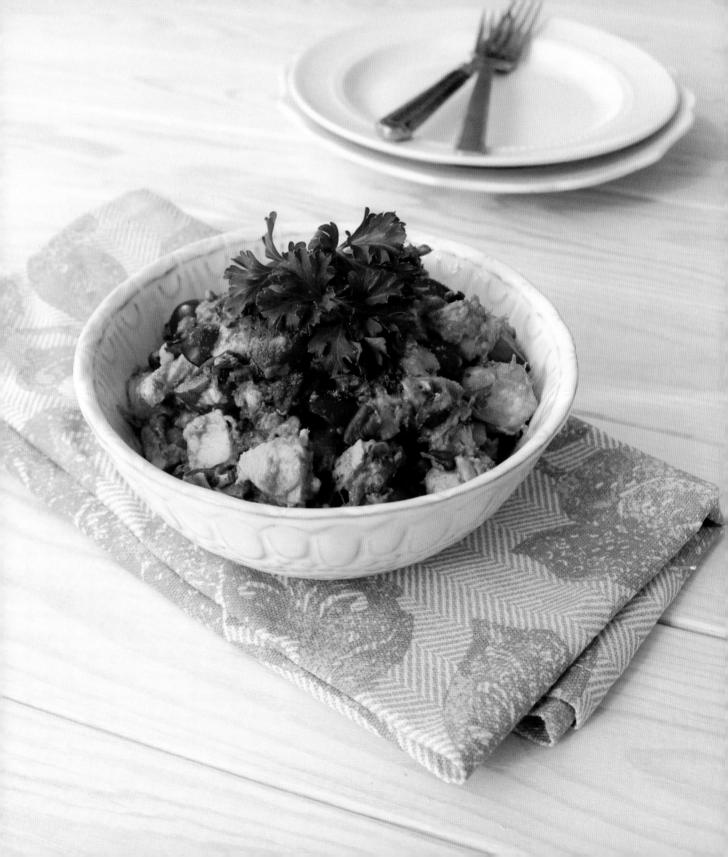

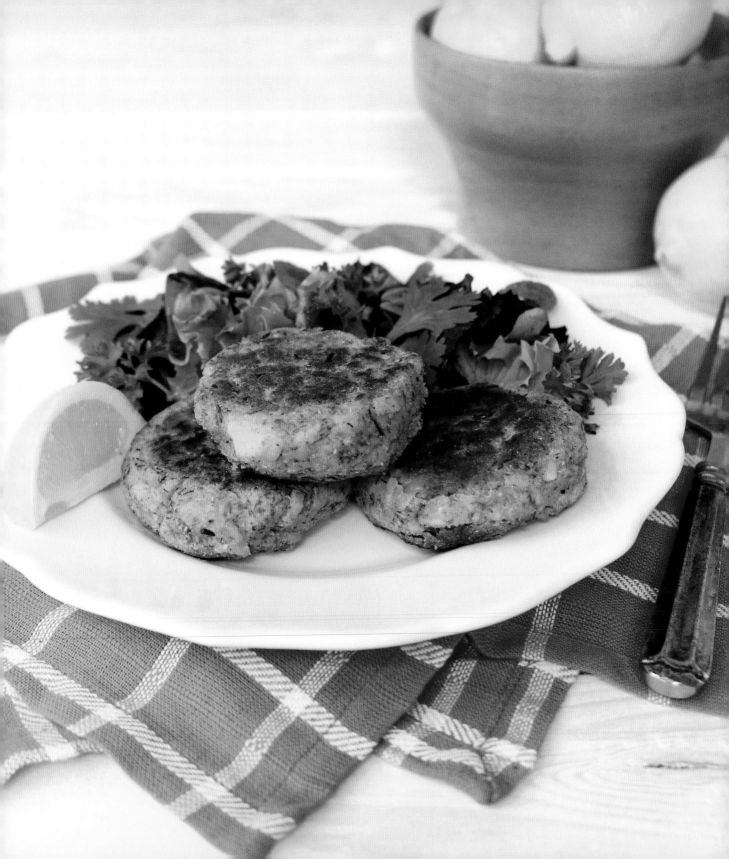

Herbed Sardine Cakes

If the word *sardine* has you instinctively pinching your nose and letting out a nasally "ewwww," then this recipe is for you. Yes, a sardine recipe just for you! I'm determined to change your mind about these little canned fish because they pack a powerful anti-inflammatory omega-3 fatty acid punch, which is critical to calming the inflammation that triggers inflammatory skin conditions and prematurely ages the skin. Plus, compared to wild salmon, sardines are super affordable and convenient—I always keep a few cans in my pantry. And I promise that you'll be pleasantly surprised at just how delicious they can be.

More glow-getting goodness: The mashed potato in this recipe provides your good gut bacteria with resistant starch, helping to maintain a healthy gut microbiome. The herbs not only add amazing flavor to the dish but also provide your skin with protective antioxidants. The eggs and avocado oil round everything out with some protein and healthy fat.

YIELD: 10 TO 12 CAKES (3 TO 4 SERVINGS)

3 medium red or white potatoes

2 large eggs

2 tbsp (18 g) coconut flour

1 tbsp (3 g) chopped fresh chives

1 tbsp (3 g) dried dill

1 tsp (1 g) dried rosemary

¼ tsp mineral-rich sea salt

12 oz (340 g) sardines in water (most cans contain 4 to 6 oz [115 to 140 g])

2 tbsp (30 ml) avocado oil

Skin and quarter the potatoes. Boil them for 15 minutes, or until they can easily be pierced with a fork. Drain, then put the potatoes in a medium mixing bowl. Mash with a fork, leaving the potatoes a little chunky. Transfer to the refrigerator to cool.

Once the potatoes have cooled, add the eggs, coconut flour, herbs and salt. Mix everything together.

Drain the sardines and place them in a separate bowl. Mash them well with a fork.

Add the sardines to the potato mixture, and mash to combine.

Using your hands, form 10 to 12 cakes 3 to 4 inches (7.5 to 10 cm) in diameter and no more than 1 inch (2.5 cm) thick.

In a large skillet over medium-low, heat the avocado oil. Make sure the bottom of the pan is covered with the oil.

Place the cakes in the oil, and cook each side for about 8 minutes, or until golden brown.

Serve with a slice of lemon and some side veggies!

Sweet and Savory Butternut Squash Chili

There's nothing quite as comforting as a big, hearty bowl of chili on a cool day. And that's exactly what this Sweet and Savory Butternut Squash Chili is: big and hearty. And of course, it's filled with skin-loving ingredients to help you get your glow on.

Butternut squash is a rich source of the antioxidants provitamin A and vitamin C, which fight age-accelerating free radicals and quell skin-irritating inflammation (refer back to page 64 for a refresher on antioxidants). It's also loaded with fiber, aiding digestion as well as hormone detoxification. Sprouted lentils are also fiber-full and a good source of protein to boot. The tomatoes and fresh spices add more skin-protecting antioxidant power. Throw everything together in a large pot and you have yourself one tasty chili that satisfies your hunger, taste buds and the skin's unique needs.

YIELD: 8 TO 10 SERVINGS

2 cups (240 g) dried sprouted lentils

1 medium butternut squash (2½ to 3 lb [1 to 1.25 kg])

2 tbsp (30 ml) avocado oil

1 large white onion, chopped

4 cups (343 g) tomato paste

½ cup (18 g) chopped fresh cilantro

2 tbsp (14 g) chili powder

1 tbsp (8 g) ground cumin

1 tsp (3 g) freshly ground black pepper

½ tsp mineral-rich sea salt

3 tbsp (45 ml) olive oil

2 cups (450 g) roughly chopped spinach

Add the lentils to a pot of 5 cups (1.2 L) of boiling water and lower the heat to medium-low. Let simmer for 5 minutes. Remove from the heat and let stand for 5 to 8 minutes.

While the lentils are cooking, chop the butternut squash: First cut the ends off and use a peeler to remove the skin. You will also need to remove the seeds.

In a large pot over medium heat, combine the avocado oil, onion and butternut squash. Stir to coat the onion and squash with the oil. Cover and let cook for 15 to 18 minutes, stirring occasionally. The squash should be tender but not too mushy.

While the squash mixture is cooking, drain the water from the lentils and return them to the pot. Add the tomato paste, 1 cup (240 ml) of water, the cilantro, chili powder, cumin, pepper, salt and olive oil to the lentils. Stir to combine.

After the onion and squash have cooked, add the spinach. Stir until the spinach is wilted.

Add the squash mixture to the lentil mixture. Stir to combine.

Simmer the chili over medium-low heat for 10 minutes.

Serve with some slices of avocado.

NOTE: Buy tomato paste that comes in a glass jar since the acids in the tomatoes readily leech hormone-disrupting plasticizers from can linings.

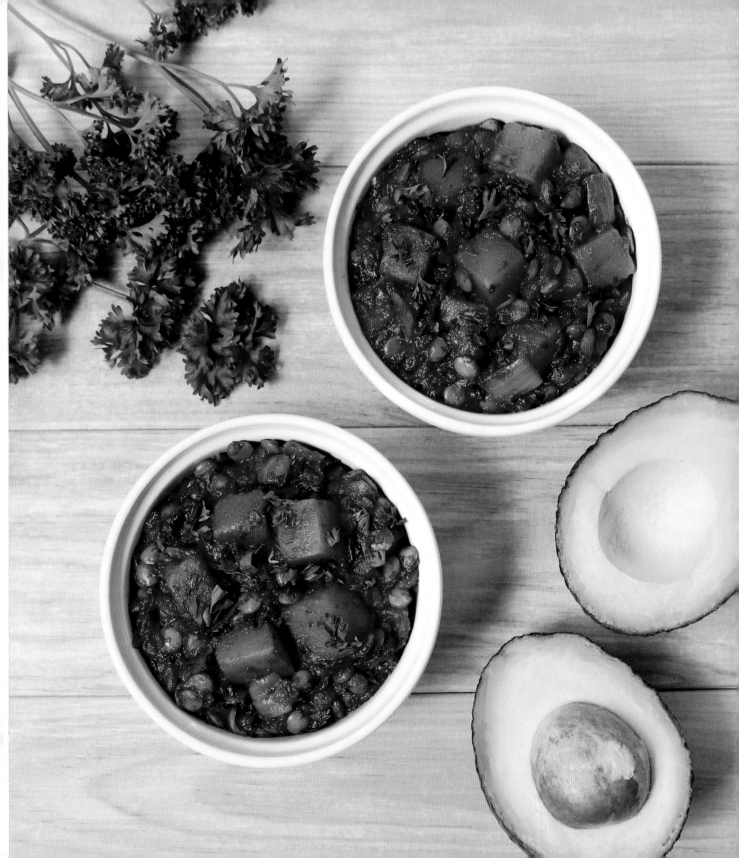

Baked "Spaghetti" Pie

Let's play a little trick on your inner carboholic. The one that says, "Pasta. I want pasta. I *need* pasta!" Oh, you know the one. This Baked "Spaghetti" Pie has the taste and feel of a traditional baked pasta, without the unhealthy insulin spike that triggers inflammatory skin conditions and disrupts collagen production (refer back to page 45 for more info)—the spaghetti squash serves as a low-glycemic, real food alternative to high-glycemic pasta, while the protein and healthy fats from the ground beef and eggs keep you satiated and blood sugar levels balanced. Plus, it's jam-packed with free radical–fighting antioxidants, especially lycopene from the tomato paste and beta-carotene from the spinach, which keep skin healthy and glowing!

YIELD: 6 TO 9 SERVINGS

1 medium spaghetti squash
(3 lb [1.5 kg])

1 yellow onion, diced

1 lb (454 g) grass-fed ground beef

2 cups (457 g) 100% tomato paste

2 cups (35 g) chopped spinach

10 sun-dried tomatoes, chopped

2 cloves garlic, peeled and minced

1 tbsp (2 g) dried basil

2 tsp (2 g) dried oregano

¼ tsp red pepper flakes

¼ tsp mineral-rich sea salt

3 large eggs, whisked

Preheat the oven to 400°F (200°C). Line a baking sheet with unbleached parchment paper. Cut off the ends of the spaghetti squash, then cut it in half widthwise. Cut the two halves widthwise again so you have 4 rounds, and remove the seeds. Set the rounds on the prepared baking sheet and bake for 25 minutes.

While the spaghetti squash is baking, cook the onion and ground beef in a large skillet or sauté pan over medium heat until the meat is fully cooked and the onion is soft. Add the tomato paste, spinach, sun-dried tomatoes, garlic, basil, oregano, red pepper flakes and salt to the meat mixture.

After the spaghetti squash has cooked, lower the oven temperature to 375°F (190°C). Let the squash cool for a few minutes so you can more easily remove the strands of "spaghetti." Using a fork, pull the strands away from the skin.

In a large bowl, mix the spaghetti squash, meat mixture and eggs together. Transfer the mixture to an 8-inch (20.5-cm) square baking dish, and bake for 45 minutes. After the pie has cooked, let it cool and set before serving.

NOTES

If you're looking to add some visual appeal to your pie, add some thinly sliced tomatoes on top before baking and garnish with fresh basil!

If you have an egg allergy or intolerance—or just want to get dinner on the table a little more quickly!—skip the eggs and final step, and simply serve the dish as you would regular old spaghetti with meat sauce.

The particular method of cooking spaghetti squash outlined here prevents it from becoming watery, which is especially important for a baked dish such as this one. No one likes watery spaghetti!

Buy your tomato paste in a glass jar since the acids in the tomatoes readily leech hormone-disrupting plasticizers from can linings.

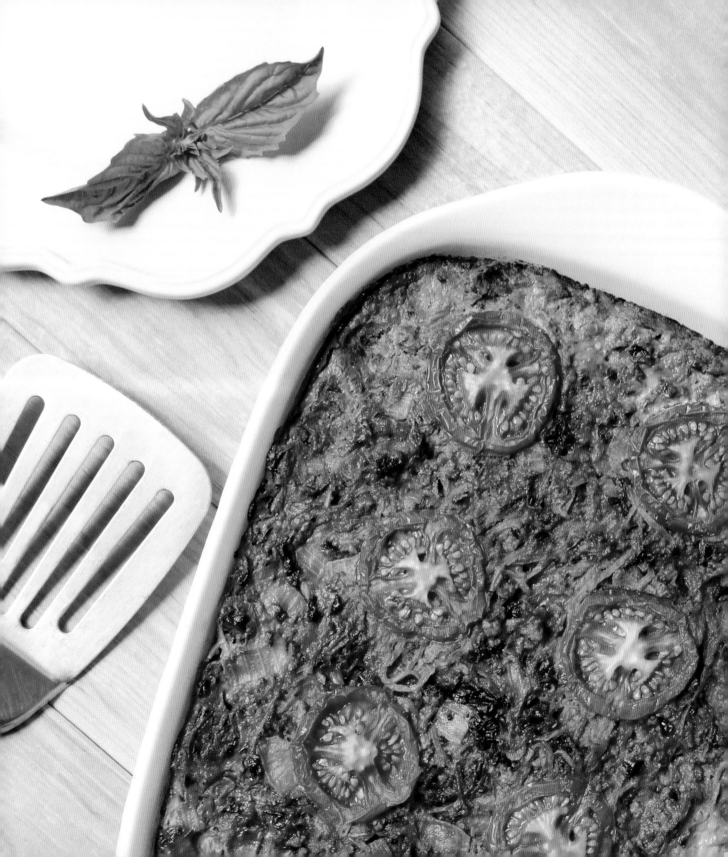

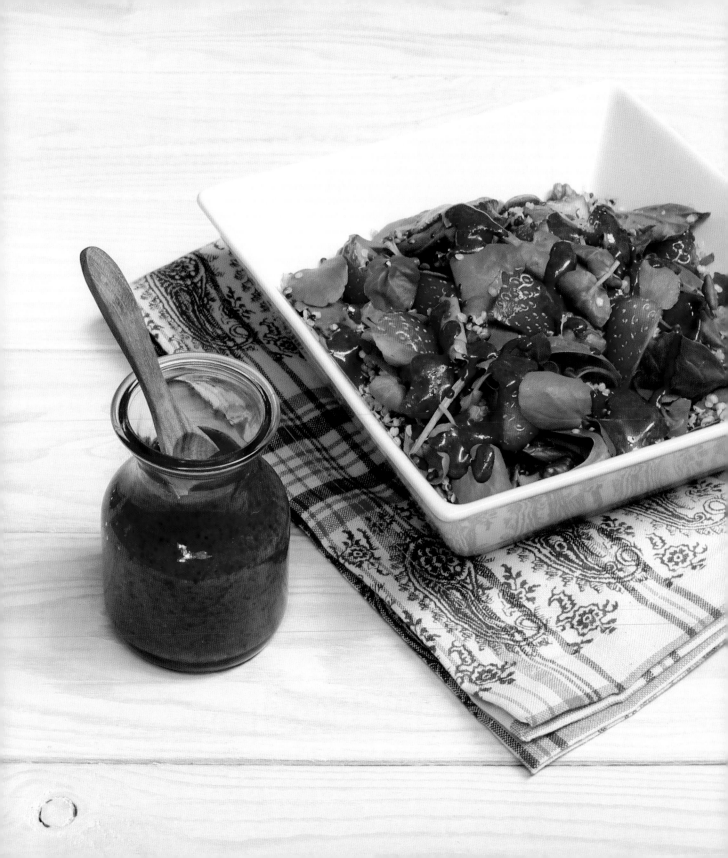

Strawberry Fields Salad with Blueberry Balsamic Dressing

This salad feels as fresh as a walk through dewy grass on a warm summer morning. Best yet, it's absolutely loaded with the skin-loving antioxidants and glow-getting nutrients necessary to build, protect and repair skin cells.

Remember, from pages 63–64, how damaging free radicals can be? Well, watercress is an antioxidant powerhouse, helping to fight off those inflammatory, DNA-damaging free radicals! Strawberries are packed with the antioxidant vitamin C, which supports collagen and elastin production, keeping skin smooth. Blueberries bring in even more antioxidant power, while olive oil provides the skin with healthy fats. Quinoa, hemp hearts and pecans bring in cell-building protein.

YIELD: 2 TO 3 SERVINGS

SALAD

½ cup (76 g) sprouted quinoa

1½ cups (52 g) watercress

1½ cups (45 g) spinach

10 fresh strawberries, sliced

¼ cup (40 g) hemp hearts

¼ cup (32 g) walnuts, crushed

DRESSING

1 cup (120 g) fresh blueberries

2 tbsp (30 ml) olive oil

2 tbsp (30 ml) balsamic vinegar

1 tsp (2 g) dried basil

½ tsp dried rosemary

⅛ tsp sea salt

Prepare the quinoa ahead of time: Add it to a pot of 1 cup (240 ml) of boiling water, then lower the heat to a simmer and cook for 7 to 9 minutes. Place in the refrigerator to cool before adding to the salad.

Place all the salad ingredients in a large salad bowl and toss to combine.

To make the dressing, in a blender or food processor, combine all the dressing ingredients. Blend until smooth and consistent.

Generously top the salad with dressing.

Sweet Pepper Mini Frittatas

As much as we may want it to, breakfast doesn't usually get first priority in the morning. That's why it's a good idea to plan ahead by making a large batch of something healthy you can grab on the go. That way you can indulge in a few extra z's or just have some quiet me-time before everyone else in the family wakes up.

These mini frittatas are the perfect glow-on-the-go breakfast—quick and easy to make ahead of time and packed with the right amounts of healthy protein and fat, which we learned are important to support the structure of the skin, balance blood sugar levels and keep you feeling full all morning. Plus, they're rich in antioxidants and vitamins, and they're oh so tasty.

YIELD: 12 MINI FRITTATAS (6 TO 8 SERVINGS)

2 tbsp (30 ml) avocado oil

1 cup (175 g) chopped red bell pepper

1 cup (175 g) chopped green bell pepper

1 cup (160 g) chopped yellow onion

¼ tsp mineral-rich sea salt

½ tsp freshly ground black pepper

2 cups (450 g) roughly chopped spinach

8 large eggs

Preheat the oven to 350°F (180°C). Grease a standard 12-cup muffin pan or line the pan with baking cups and set aside.

Heat a large skillet over medium heat.

Once the skillet is hot, add the avocado oil, red pepper, green pepper and onion. Sauté for 5 to 7 minutes, or until the peppers are tender.

Add the salt, black pepper and spinach to the skillet and sauté for an additional 2 minutes.

Crack the eggs into a large mixing bowl and whisk together.

Add the cooked veggies to the eggs and mix together.

Pour the mixture evenly into the prepared muffin cups.

Bake for 18 to 20 minutes, or until the tops of the frittatas are firm to the touch and the eggs are cooked.

Either serve immediately or store in the refrigerator for up to 5 days to be enjoyed as a glow-getting on-the-go breakfast at a later date!

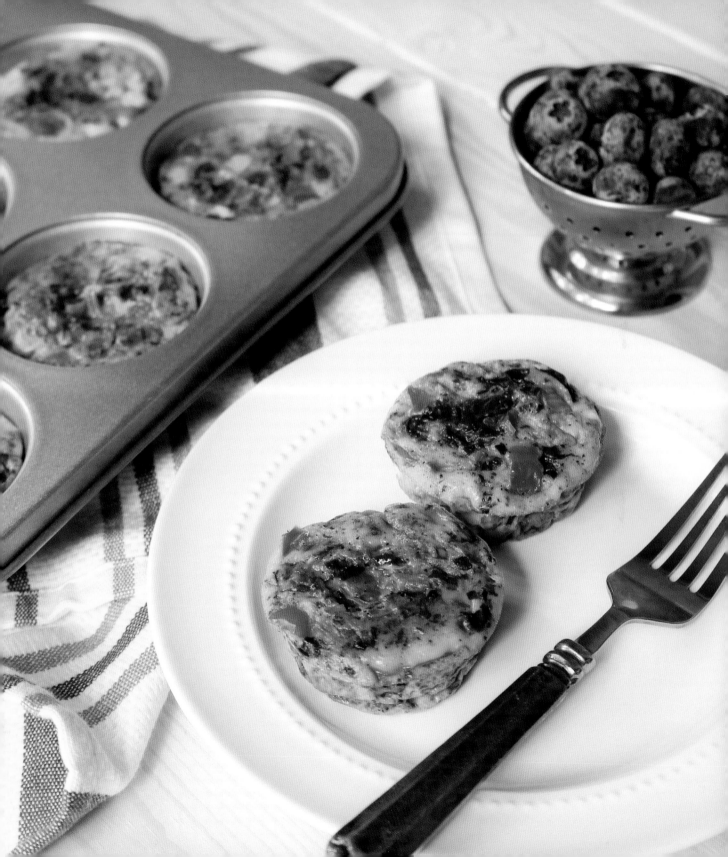

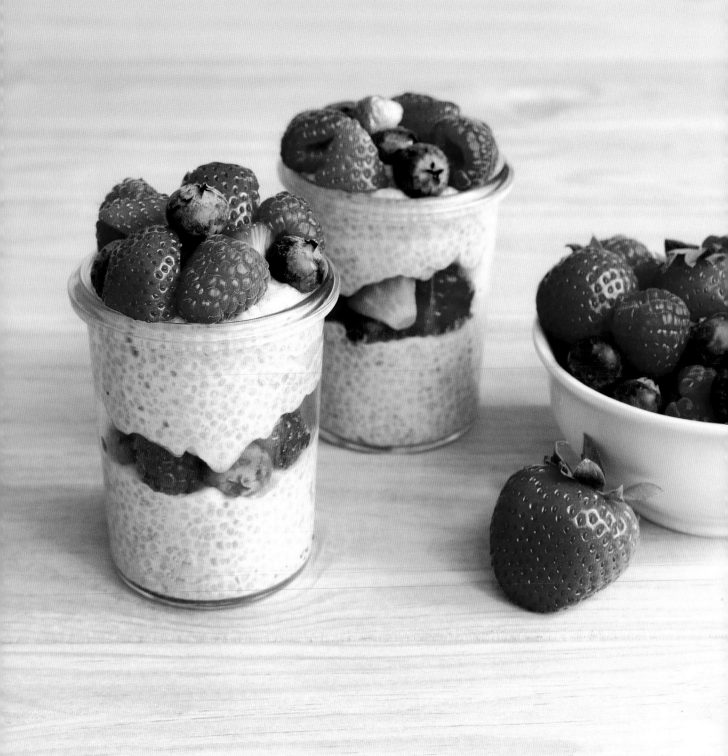

Berry Satisfying Chia Pudding Parfait

If you haven't jumped on the chia pudding train yet, consider this your formal invitation to come aboard. This recipe is a twist on the classic, with even more skin-loving ingredients included.

Chia seeds are a good source of the anti-inflammatory omega-3 fatty acids as well as cleansing fiber. The healthy fats in chia seeds and coconut milk maintain healthy skin cells and keep you feeling full. Collagen peptides provide all of the skin-building amino acids plus protein to help keep you feeling satiated, which, you'll recall from page 28, is extremely important for maintaining steady blood sugar levels. Add the antioxidant power of blueberries and strawberries and you've got yourself one delicious, glow-getting breakfast.

YIELD: 2 SERVINGS

1 cup (240 ml) coconut milk (for homemade, see page 120)

1 tsp (5 ml) pure vanilla extract

¼ cup (22 g) collagen peptides

¼ cup (48 g) chia seeds

½ cup (40 g) fresh berries

In a medium bowl, combine the coconut milk, vanilla and collagen peptides and stir. Add the chia seeds and stir.

Let the mixture sit for a couple of minutes, during which time the chia seeds will begin to absorb the liquid and expand, then stir again.

Place the pudding in the refrigerator to set for another 10 minutes.

To create parfaits, layer the chia pudding and berries in two glasses or jars (this recipe fits perfectly in two 8-ounce [240-ml] mason jars).

Eat immediately or store in the refrigerator for up to 4 days to be enjoyed at a later date as a healthy, glow-on-the-go breakfast!

Nadia's Go-to Green Smoothie

Smoothies are the ultimate fast food: Throw everything in a blender, pour in a mason jar and go! This particular recipe is my favorite—I drink it almost every day as a quick, glow-on-the-go meal.

As we discussed back on page 31, monounsaturated fatty acids, such as those abundant in avocados, are extremely skin-supportive, helping to maintain healthy cell membranes and proper moisture balance. Pineapple lends sweetness as well as anti-inflammatory enzymes. Kale and spinach feed skin with a host of vitamins and minerals, while collagen peptides and bee propolis each provide your skin with supportive amino acids.

YIELD: 20 OZ (625 ML)

½ avocado

½ banana

¼ cup (20 g) frozen chopped spinach

¼ cup (21 g) frozen kale

5 chunks frozen pineapple

2 tbsp (11 g) collagen peptides

1 tsp (5 g) bee propolis

1½ cups (360 ml) coconut milk
(for homemade, see page 120)

In a blender, combine all the ingredients and blend on high speed until smooth and consistent.

Like I said, fast food!

NOTE: I use frozen ingredients to save me both some time and money—not only are frozen spinach, kale and pineapple already cut for me, they're most often cheaper than their fresh counterparts and just as nutritious (in fact, some studies have found that frozen produce is more nutritious since it's flash frozen soon after being harvested, when it is most nutrient-dense). Plus, with frozen produce, you're sure to always have the ingredients on hand and don't have to worry about spoiling!

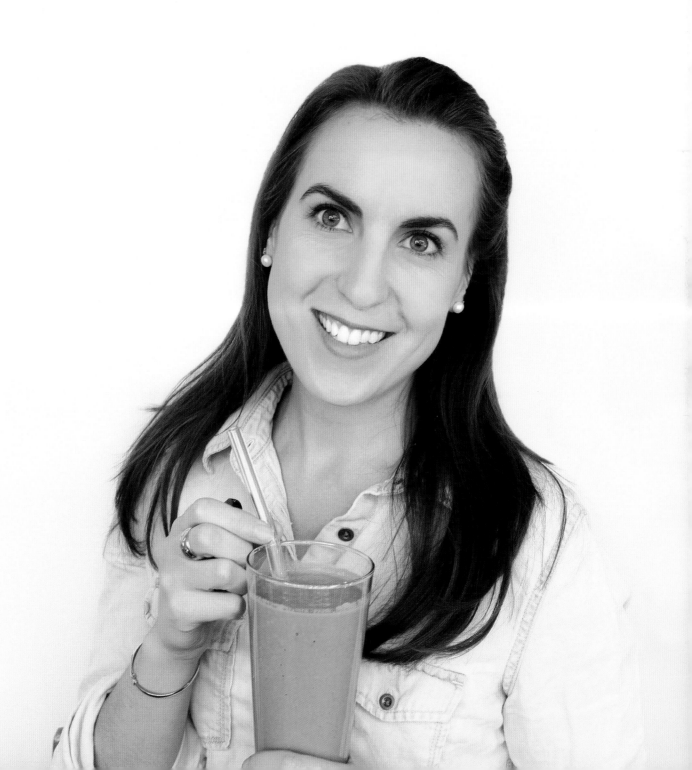

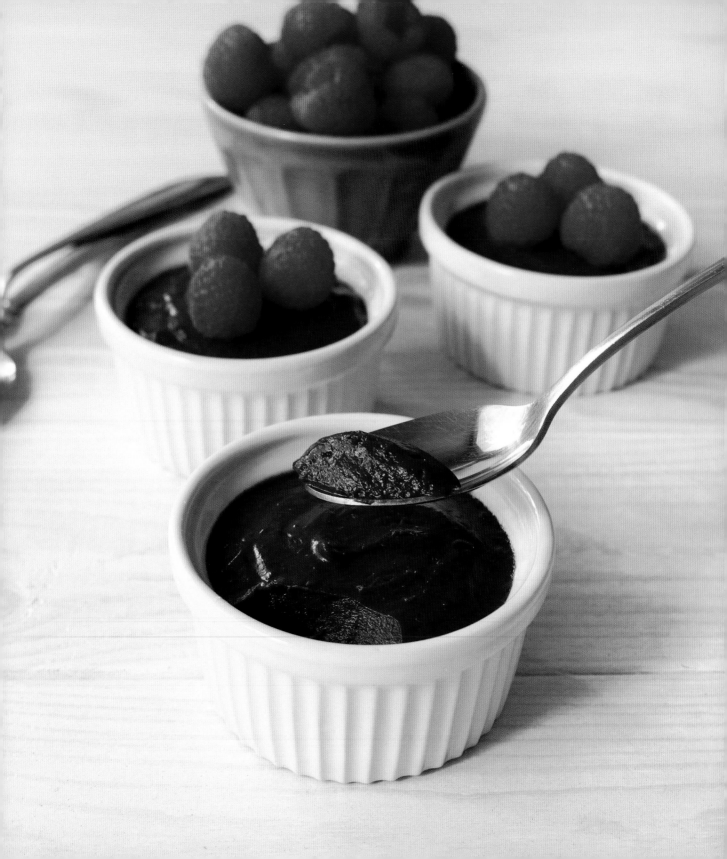

AvoCacao Pot de Crème

Are you a chocolate lover? A fan of chocolate cake filled with chocolate ganache topped with a warm chocolate drizzle? Well then, this is the glow-getting treat for you.

This AvoCacao Pot de Crème is incredibly rich, smooth and satisfying. With a base of avocado (though each of my guinea pigs couldn't guess it!), it's filled with skin-supporting healthy fats, fiber, vitamin E and a number of the B family members. Raw cacao powder protects skin with antioxidants, fighting free radicals and reducing inflammation. Although it contains raw honey for added sweetness, the fiber and healthy fats from the avocado and coconut oil help to temper the effect on blood sugar, making this a healthy option for your sweet tooth!

YIELD: 2 TO 3 SERVINGS

2 avocados

3 tbsp (45 ml) raw honey

3 tbsp (42 g) extra-virgin coconut oil

4 tbsp (56 g) raw cacao powder

1 tsp (5 ml) pure vanilla extract

Pinch of mineral-rich sea salt

Peel and pit the avocados.

In a medium mixing bowl, mash the avocados with a fork.

Add the raw honey and coconut oil. Stir to combine, but don't worry about consistency.

Add the cacao powder and stir to combine.

Transfer the mixture to a blender or food processor and add the vanilla. Blend or process on low speed until you have a smooth and consistent pudding texture.

Pour the mixture into a bowl or small ramekins and let chill in the refrigerator for at least 30 minutes so it has time to set.

Sprinkle with the sea salt just before serving.

NOTE: Even though this pudding is made with healthy, real food ingredients, it still contains quite a bit of sugar from the raw honey. So, try not to go crazy with it! Keep in mind that this recipe makes 2 to 3 servings, and treat it as such.

Sweet Roots Sauerkraut

This ain't your grandma's sauerkraut (though, don't get me wrong, I'm sure it was quite delicious). This kraut has a sweet and zesty twist, thanks to its all-star cast of skin-loving ingredients. It's also very simple to make and costs just a fraction of what the fresh ferments in the refrigerated section of the health food store do.

Fermented foods are a fantastic source of probiotics, which not only aid digestion but also keep the gut in tip-top shape. Cabbage is high in the antioxidant glutamine, which helps build the mucus layer that protects the gut. Remember, from page 49, that the gut and skin are considered "two sides of the same coin," so when the gut is happy, it shows on the skin. Carrots, beets and ginger bring in antioxidants and glow-getting vitamins. Beets are also a liver-loving superfood, helping the digestion of healthy fats and hormone balance, two more keys to glowing skin from within! Enjoy a couple of tablespoons of this kraut as a snack or with a meal for a glow-getting boost of goodness.

YIELD: 2 CUPS (367 G)

2 cups (100 g) chopped red cabbage

1 cup (160 g) coarsely grated beet

1 cup (90 g) coarsely grated carrot

2 tsp (4 g) finely grated fresh ginger

1 tbsp (6 g) orange zest

1¼ tsp (7 g) mineral-rich sea salt

1 whole cabbage leaf

In a superclean mixing bowl, combine the red cabbage, beet, carrot, ginger and orange zest. Sprinkle the salt on top.

With clean hands, massage the salt into the mixture.

Transfer the mixture (including any juices) to a clean mason jar, and pack with a clean spoon. Cover the top of the mixture with a cabbage leaf and pack it down again. Cover the jar with a clean cloth and secure it with a rubber band.

After 24 hours, take a peek at how things are progressing. Pack everything down again with a clean spoon. If the liquid is not covering the top of the solids, mix ½ teaspoon of salt with ½ cup (120 ml) of water and add *just* enough to bring the liquid level to the top of the solid mixture.

Let the mixture sit on the counter for 2 to 7 more days. Keep an eye on it during this time: Skim any floating scum from the surface (it's supposed to be there—don't let it scare you!) and use a clean spoon to press down any of the solid mixture that floats above the liquid. There is no "rule" for when sauerkraut is done fermenting. After 3 days, taste a sample of your kraut each day—when it tastes good to you, it's done!

After your sauerkraut is done fermenting (i.e., it's been sitting for at least 3 days and tastes good to you), transfer it to the refrigerator.

Enjoy a few tablespoons with or between meals!

Best if consumed within 1 month.

NOTES

Notice how I mentioned cleanliness quite a bit? Well, while we want the healthy bacteria from the cabbage, beet and carrot to grow, we don't want any unhealthy bacteria to do so.

Take care when grating the beet! Beet juice stains, so be careful not to let it get on your clothing or sit on porous countertops for too long.

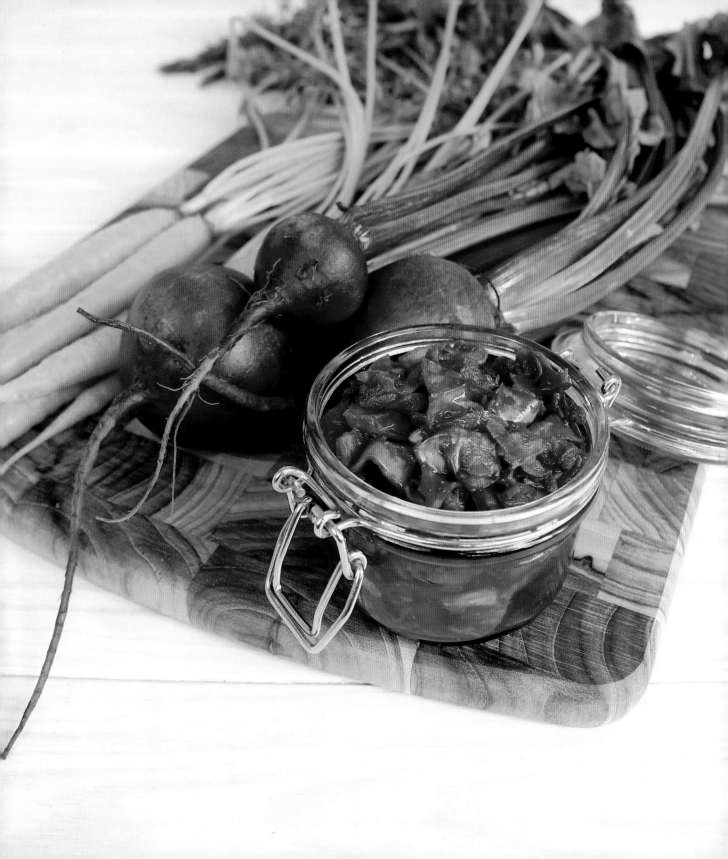

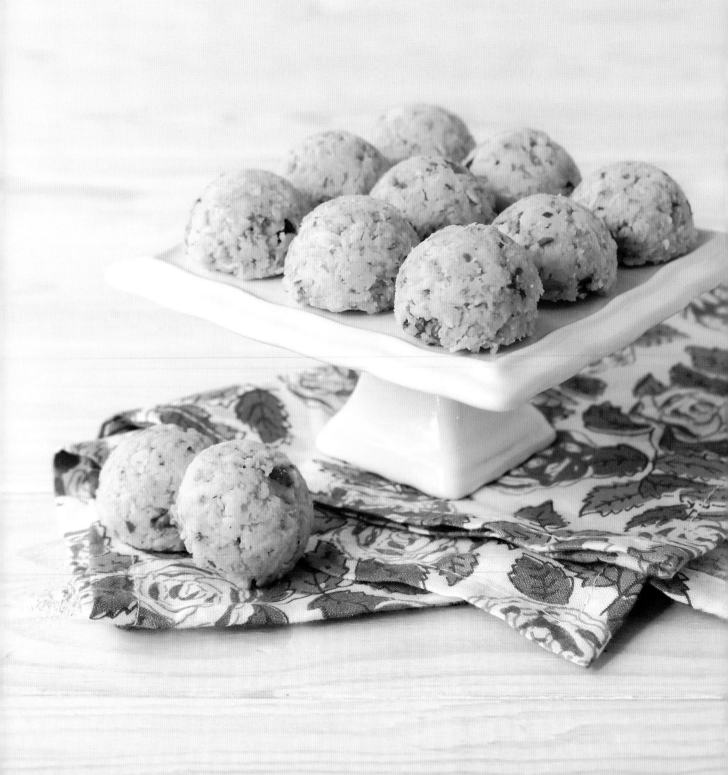

Coconutty Energy Bites

When you start to feel a hankering for something naughty and skin-unfriendly, reach for these Coconutty Energy Bites. They're subtly sweet yet loaded with healthy fats to keep you feeling full and satiated—the ultimate cure for cravings.

Healthy fats are also vital for healthy, supple, glowing skin. The flaxseeds and walnuts provide omega-3 fatty acids, which help to fight the skin-irritating inflammation behind pesky skin issues like acne and eczema as well as premature aging.

YIELD: 25 (½-TBSP [15-G]) BITES

¾ cup (192 g) coconut butter

2 tbsp (30 ml) pure maple syrup

½ cup (48 g) unsweetened shredded coconut

½ cup (45 g) gluten-free rolled oats

¼ cup (28 g) ground flaxseed

⅓ cup (40 g) chopped walnuts

¼ tsp mineral-rich sea salt

If the coconut butter is solid: Place an oven-safe liquid measuring cup in a small pot filled with shallow, boiling water, and scoop the coconut butter into the measuring cup. Keep adding coconut butter until it reaches the ¾-cup (180-ml) measurement.

In a large mixing bowl, combine all the ingredients.

Place the mixture in the refrigerator for 10 to 15 minutes so it will firm up a bit (this will make it easier to form into bites).

Once the mixture has cooled slightly, form the bites using your hands or a ½-tablespoon (7.5-g) cookie scoop (be sure to push the mixture into the scoop to compact it).

These will keep in the refrigerator for up to 5 days.

> **NOTE:** If you'd rather save the time and keep from getting your hands dirty, you can simply press the mixture into a baking dish lined with parchment paper, set it into the refrigerator to cool and then cut it into bars.

Spiced Sweet Potato Muffins

Mmm, a hot, Spiced Sweet Potato Muffin with some tea . . . this is a lovely way to unwind after a long day or take a midday siesta, even if just for 3 minutes at your desk between meetings. Not only are these muffins delicious, they're jam-packed with nutrients to help you get your glow on while keeping you feeling full and satiated.

Sweet potato is a rich source of the antioxidants provitamin A and vitamin C, which we know protect skin from free radical damage and fight skin-irritating inflammation. It's also loaded with fiber, aiding digestion as well as hormone detoxification. The eggs not only provide a ton of glow-getting nutrients, but their protein and fat keeps you full and slows glucose absorption to prevent an inflammatory, skin-sabotaging insulin spike.

YIELD: 8 MUFFINS

1 large sweet potato

5 large eggs

3 tbsp (45 ml) pure maple syrup

2 tsp (10 ml) pure vanilla extract

2 tsp (5 g) ground cinnamon

½ tsp freshly grated nutmeg

½ tsp ground ginger

⅛ tsp mineral-rich sea salt

½ cup (144 g) coconut flour

Preheat the oven to 400°F (200°C). Wash the sweet potato and pierce it 8 to 10 times with a fork.

Place the sweet potato on a cookie sheet or in a baking dish and bake for 45 to 50 minutes. When it is done cooking, the outside will have darkened and the inside will be soft. Set the sweet potato aside to cool.

Lower the oven to 350°F (180°C). Grease 8 cups of a standard 12-cup muffin pan or line the pan with baking cups and set aside.

Measure out 1 cup (250 g) of baked sweet potato and transfer to a blender.

Add the eggs, maple syrup, vanilla, cinnamon, nutmeg, ginger and sea salt. Blend on low speed for a minute to create a consistent batter.

Add the coconut flour to the batter, and blend on low speed for another minute to combine. If necessary, push down the batter with a spatula.

Scoop the batter into the prepared muffin cups.

Bake for 22 to 25 minutes.

Either consume right away or store in the fridge for a glow-on-the-go treat later!

NOTE: I typically bake quite a few sweet potatoes at once and keep the others for a snack or quick side dish option! That way, I'm not running the oven for so long for just one little potato.

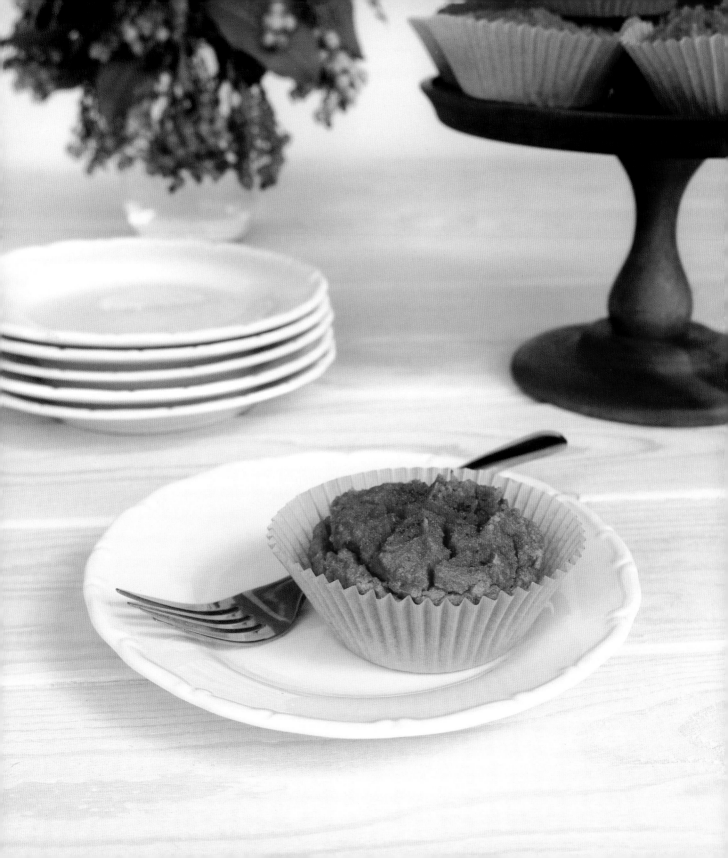

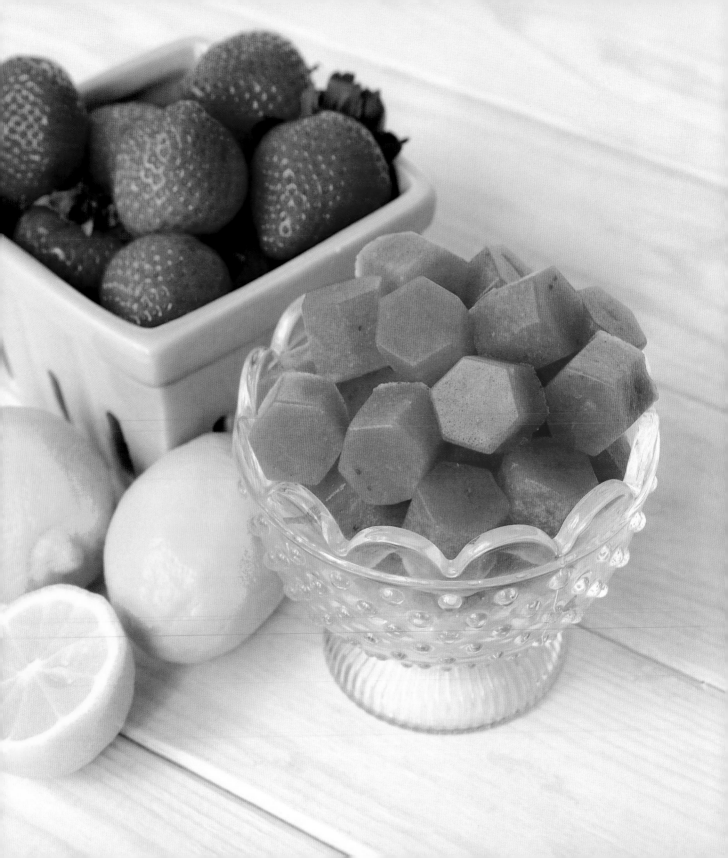

Strawberry Lemonade Fruit Snacks

Chewy fruit snacks have a very special place in my heart. They're just so fun to eat and remind me of being a kid! While most store-bought fruit snacks are filled with unhealthy ingredients that certainly do not bode well for the skin, these homemade Strawberry Lemonade Fruit Snacks help support healthy skin from the inside out.

Strawberries and lemons are both rich in the antioxidant vitamin C, which we learned fights aging and inflammatory free radicals. As highlighted on page 28, grass-fed gelatin provides the skin with all of the amino acids it needs to build strong, healthy cells, particularly supporting collagen and elastin production. It's also a gut-healing superfood, helping to remedy this common skin trigger.

YIELD: 1¼ CUPS (285 ML)

⅔ cup (160 ml) freshly squeezed lemon juice

1 cup (164 g) sliced strawberries

6 drops liquid stevia extract

4 tbsp (22 g) gelatin

In a high-speed blender, combine the lemon juice, strawberries and stevia extract and blend on high speed for 30 seconds.

Continue to blend on the lowest speed and slowly add the gelatin 1 tablespoon (5 g) at a time (at such a low speed, you shouldn't have to worry about the mixture splashing up out of the blender and making a mess). Blend for just 5 more seconds after the last tablespoon (5 g) of gelatin has been added to the mixture.

Quickly transfer the mixture to a small pot over medium heat. Stir the mixture consistently for about 2 minutes, or until it is just warmer than body temperature.

Pour the mixture into silicone candy molds or a glass-baking dish.

Place the candy molds or baking dish in the refrigerator to set for an hour.

After setting for an hour in the refrigerator, either pop the fruit snacks out of the molds or slice the gelatin mixture in the baking dish into bite-size squares.

Store in the refrigerator for up to 4 days.

NOTE: If you prefer your fruit snacks sourer, omit the stevia extract.

Tropical Turmeric Ice Pops

Not only are these ice pops a yummy taste of the tropics, they contain two anti-inflammatory powerhouses—pineapple and turmeric—to deliciously help fight the inflammation that we learned can be so damaging to the skin. They're also packed with the skin-loving vitamins A and C, thanks to the mango and orange juice. And since the curcumin in turmeric is fat-soluble, we want to pair it with healthy fats such as those from coconut and avocado, which also help to keep blood sugar levels from spiking.

YIELD: ABOUT 12 OZ (340 G), OR 4 POPS (DEPENDING ON YOUR SPECIFIC MOLDS)

1 cup (165 g) fresh mango chunks

1 cup (245 g) fresh pineapple chunks

½ cup (120 ml) fresh orange juice
(from about 1 orange)

¼ cup (56 g) coconut manna

½ avocado

2 tsp (6 g) organic ground turmeric or
1 inch (2.5 cm) of peeled turmeric root

In a blender, combine all the ingredients and blend until smooth.

Transfer the mixture to your ice pop molds and freeze for at least 2 hours.

Store in the freezer until you're ready to enjoy them!

NOTES

You can certainly use frozen mango and pineapple chunks, but let them thaw beforehand so they will blend easily.

To add some visual appeal to your pops, roll them in shredded coconut before serving!

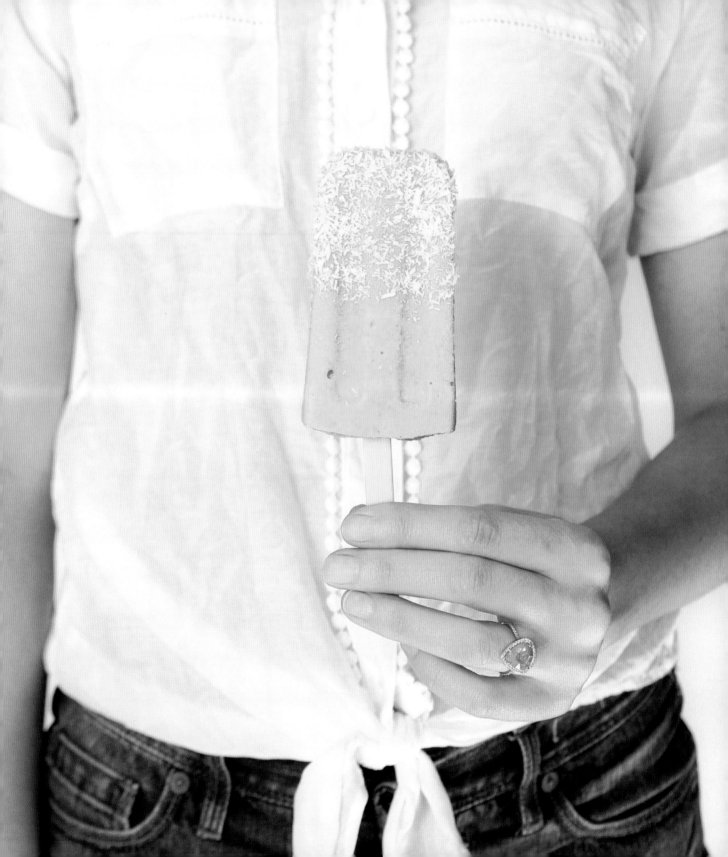

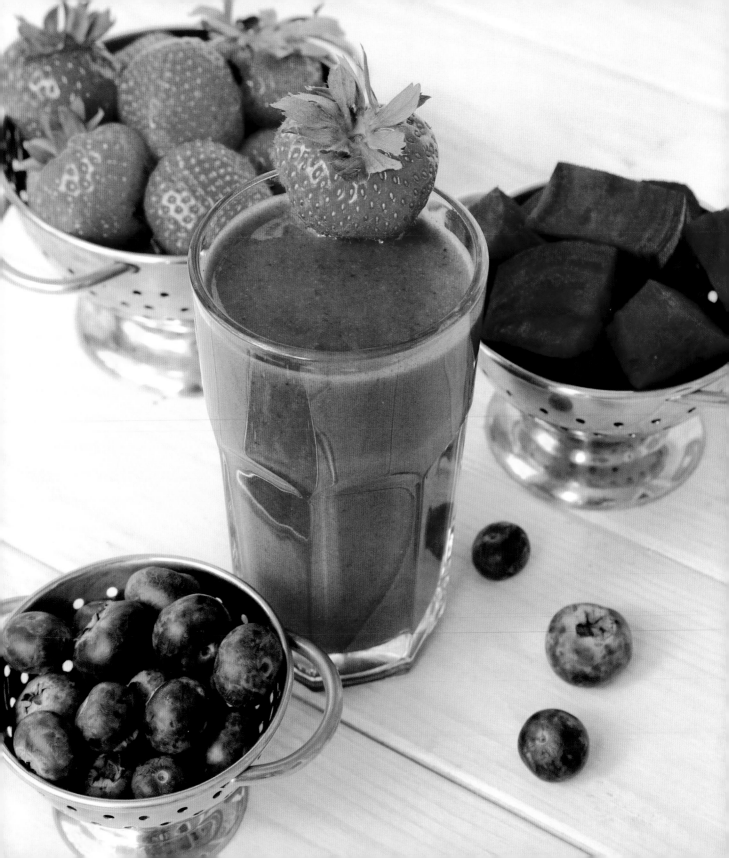

Beet and Berry Smoothie

If you've never quite been able to get on team beet, I triple dog dare you to try this Beet and Berry Smoothie. Because not only do berries and beets unite to form one powerhouse antioxidant combo, they're darn delicious together, too!

The antioxidants in this smoothie help fight free radicals and inflammation, slowing aging and quelling inflammatory skin issues. In addition to their rich antioxidant content, beets are also a liver-loving superfood, helping this vital organ detox potentially skin-harming toxins and excess hormones. The avocado and coconut oil provide healthy fats to keep the skin glowing, the tummy satisfied and the smoothie creamy. Protein-packed collagen peptides add extra sustenance and skin-loving goodness, making this smoothie the complete package.

YIELD: 20 OZ (590 ML) (SERVES 2)

½ avocado

½ cup (65 g) diced beet

½ cup (50 g) frozen blueberries

4 strawberries, hulled (48 g)

1½ cups (360 ml) coconut milk
(for homemade, see page 120)

In a high-speed blender, combine all the ingredients. Blend on high speed for 1 to 2 minutes, or until the texture is smooth and consistent.

NOTE: Since this smoothie is rather high in natural sugars, I consider it to be a treat rather than a meal. The 20 ounce (625 ml) smoothie is best split into 2 servings.

Good Morning Anti-Inflammatory Elixir

Having a healthy morning routine gets you off on the right foot, setting a positive tone for the day ahead. And what better way to begin your day than with the glow-getting goodness of this anti-inflammatory elixir?

Starting the day with a large glass of water helps hydrate the body, which is important in and of itself. Mineral-rich sea salt aids hydration by providing your body with electrolytes. Apple cider vinegar and fresh lemon juice jump-start the digestive system by stimulating the secretion of gastric juices, helping to ensure that your healthy breakfast will be appropriately digested so your skin can access all of those glow-getting nutrients. The antioxidant vitamin C in lemon juice gives the liver a helping hand and protects the skin from inflammatory free radicals. Last but certainly not least, turmeric and ginger contain potent anti-inflammatory compounds, fighting skin-irritating inflammation.

YIELD: 12 OZ (355 ML)

1½ cups (360 ml) warm water
(just above body temperature)

½ lemon

1 tsp (5 ml) apple cider vinegar

1 tsp (5 ml) raw honey

⅛ tsp ground turmeric

⅛ tsp ground ginger

Pinch of mineral-rich sea salt

Juice the lemon directly into the glass of warm water.

Add the vinegar, honey, turmeric, ginger and sea salt to the water, and stir to combine.

Bottoms up!

NOTES

Drinking through a straw will prevent the acids from the lemon and vinegar from damaging your tooth enamel. If you make this elixir part of your daily routine, invest in some glass or stainless-steel straws!

After drinking this morning elixir, wait 10 to 15 minutes before having breakfast, to allow the water to leave your stomach and the vinegar ample time to stimulate your gastric juices.

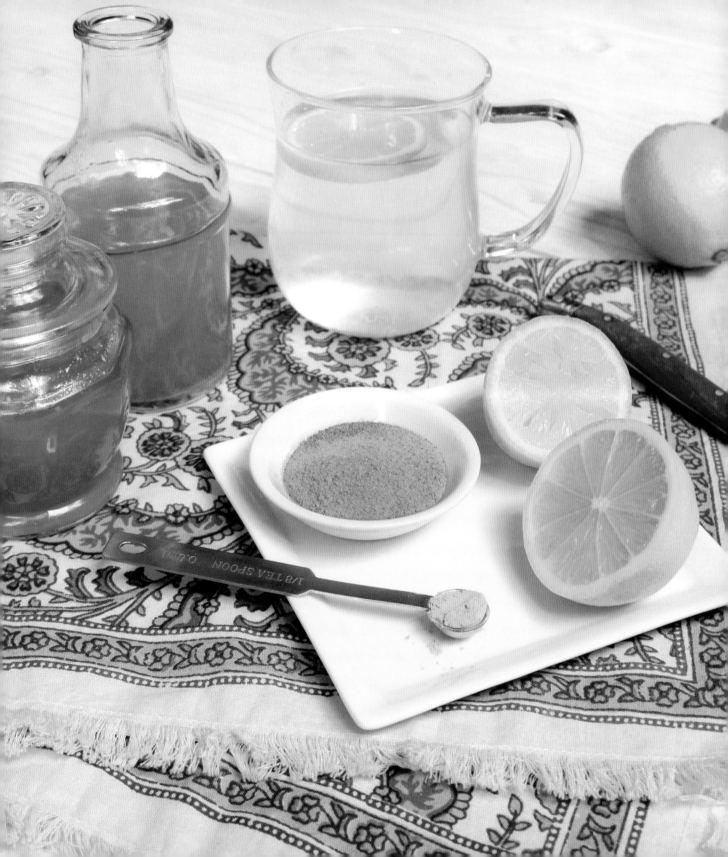

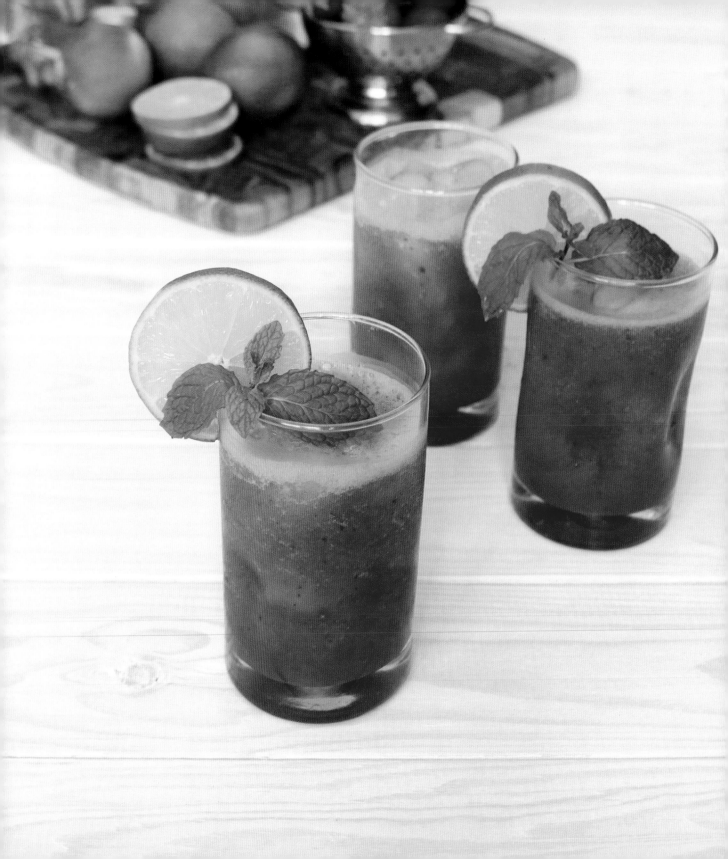

"Hello Sunshine" Juice

This ridiculously yummy juice is meant for sipping poolside or by the surf. Not only will it have your taste buds rejoicing, "Summer is here!" but its powerhouse ingredients help protect skin from the damaging effects of UV rays, which promote premature aging, damage cell DNA and oxidize sebum.

Both the lycopene in tomatoes and the catechins in green tea have been shown to protect skin from UV rays by neutralizing free radicals. The vitamin C in lime juice and strawberries provides antioxidant protection as well, and also protects the green tea's delicate antioxidants, making them even more powerful.

YIELD: 4½ CUPS (ABOUT 1.1 L) (4 TO 5 SERVINGS)

1 tbsp (2 g) loose green tea, or 3 green tea bags

1½ cups (360 ml) hot (not quite boiling) water

1 lb (454 g) fresh seedless watermelon

½ cup (120 ml) freshly squeezed lime juice

8 strawberries, hulled

4 large mint leaves

Brew a strong cup of green tea by pouring the hot water over the tea. Let the tea steep for 3 minutes (any longer and it will be bitter), then strain out the leaves or remove the tea bags. Put the tea in the refrigerator to cool.

In a high-speed blender, puree the watermelon, adding the fruit until the juice reaches the 2-cup (480-ml) marker on the blender.

Once the green tea has cooled, add it to the watermelon puree in the blender along with the lime juice, strawberries and mint leaves. Blend to combine.

Serve over ice.

Simple Homemade Coconut Milk

Whether or not you've cut dairy from your diet, a trusty and yummy nondairy milk is a staple ingredient to always have on hand. Making your own is so super simple and very cost effective, as well as a great way to avoid unnecessary (and sometimes unhealthy) thickeners and emulsifiers commonly found in store-bought nondairy milks.

Coconut milk is undoubtedly one of the healthiest nondairy milk options. As highlighted on page 34, coconut fat is filled with metabolism-boosting and nourishing MCTs. Its antibacterial properties have been shown to improve the immune system and keep the gut microbiome in balance, keeping the skin healthy and glowing.

Remember: If you have acne, a food intolerance to dairy or you're not able to buy quality, grass-fed raw or organic dairy products, dairy shouldn't be on the menu. This coconut milk is a great alternative.

YIELD: 4 CUPS (960 ML)

4 cups (960 ml) filtered water

2½ cups (240 g) unsweetened shredded coconut

In a blender, combine the water and shredded coconut and blend on high speed for 30 seconds to 1 minute. Transfer the mixture to a pot, place over medium heat and heat until it is hot but not boiling. Then, turn off the burner and allow the mixture to cool for about half an hour.

Finally, position a nut milk bag in a large bowl so that you can pour the mixture into the bag. Pour the mixture into the bag, and wring the milk out of the bag—the coconut pulp will be left behind in the bag.

Bottle your coconut milk and enjoy it within 5 days!

NOTES

A tablespoon (15 ml) of pure vanilla extract and a few drops of pure liquid stevia extract are a great way to add some extra favor and a bit of natural sweetness to your coconut milk.

The fat in the coconut milk will separate from the water. Simply shake it up before using.

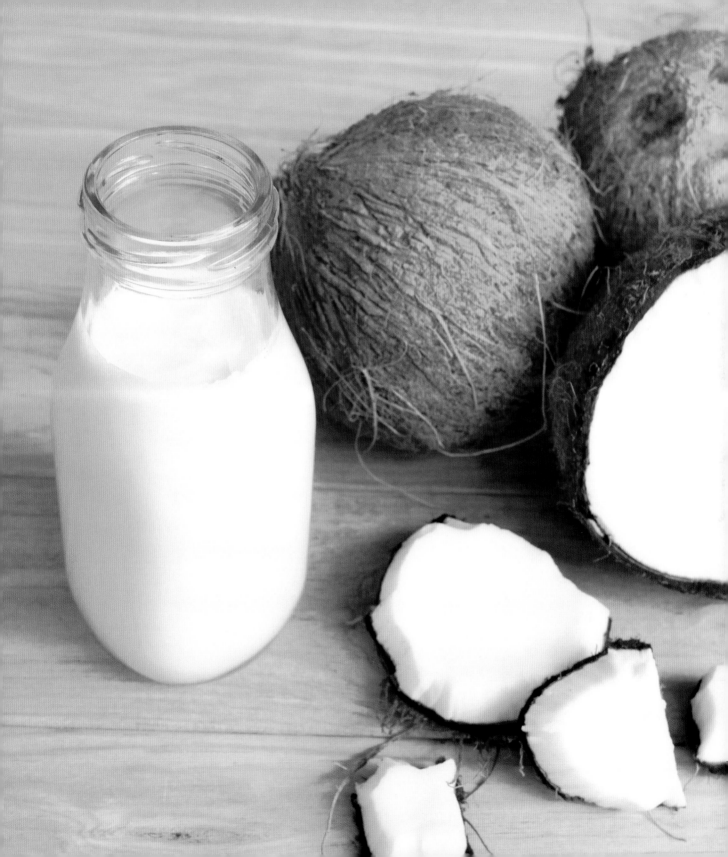

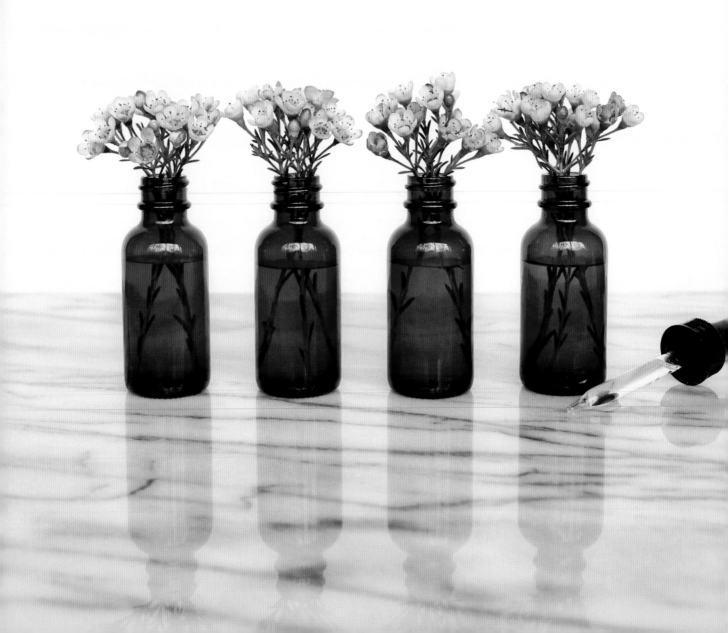

Boost Your Inner Glow

· · ·

DETOX YOUR SKINCARE ROUTINE

IT'S TIME TO CLEAN UP YOUR ACT

Your mama was wrong: beauty is not only skin deep.

We're now well aware of the many ways in which the skin is impacted by everything happening below our skin, in our bodies. But what about the other way around? Can what we apply to our skin impact what is happening in our bodies? The answer is yes.

The skin is a sponge that soaks up the majority of what we put on it. (Think about it for a moment: The efficacy of transdermal medications, such as birth control and nicotine patches, depends on this fact.) Unfortunately, most common skincare products are filled with unhealthy chemicals.

Most of us don't ever consider the ingredients in our cosmetic products. I, for one, always thought that if something was for sale, it must be safe. I mean, it wouldn't otherwise be allowed for sale, right? Unfortunately, that's just not the case—beauty and personal care products are a primary source of our chemical exposure.

On the average day, the average woman wears hundreds of chemicals. These chemicals are found in her face wash, face lotion, toner, shampoo, body lotion, deodorant, perfume, mascara, eye shadow, foundation . . . and so the list goes on and on. Most of these have not been well studied for safety, and of those that have, a number show significant cause for concern.

Here's the real kicker: These chemicals really don't do anything safer, natural ingredients can't! I've had this discussion with numerous friends and readers. They say something like, "With all of these new lines starting to show, I feel like I really *need* those chemicals." But Mother Nature's gifts know no bounds. Just as vitamins, minerals, fatty acids, phytonutrients and antioxidants keep our bodies healthy and skin glowing from the inside, they also work wonders for the skin from the outside.

Simple, natural ingredients, such as oils, butters and herbs are bursting with these skin-loving goodies. Plus, most store-bought, conventional skincare products aren't much more than a small amount of active ingredient, water, thickeners and preservatives. Most natural products, on the other hand— especially the ones you make yourself—are bursting with effective ingredients that each work to nourish, perfect and protect your skin.

When it comes to detoxing your skincare routine, it's a matter of:

1. Understanding why it is so important to avoid exposure to unhealthy chemicals in skincare products

2. Getting acquainted with some of the unhealthy chemicals most commonly used in skincare products

3. Learning about safer skincare options

4. Opening up to the world of DIY skincare

At first, it's difficult to understand how something as seemingly innocent as face wash or body lotion could possibly pose a significant threat to your health.

After all, you use such a small amount!

But here's the thing: We may use a small amount of these products, but we use them every day and sometimes multiple times a day. So, what we have is low-grade, chronic exposure to these chemicals.

Many of these chemicals have been directly or indirectly linked to hormone disruption, DNA damage and even cancer. Even more concerning: The majority of the chemicals in use have never even been studied. More concerning *still* is that companies are able to keep some chemicals a secret as trade secrets. So, we may not even know everything that is actually in a product!

While some of these chemicals are detoxed from the body quickly, others bioaccumulate, meaning they make a nice little cozy home in our fat cells where they may live until the day we die. And while these chemicals are hanging out in our bodies, they may meet one another and become friends. And who knows what could result of this friendship? They may hold hands and sing "Kumbaya" or join forces and raise hell—there is a very legitimate concern that these chemicals could react once in our body, resulting in who-knows-what sort of new chemical and cause harm. This is a huge unknown, of course. But I know one thing for sure: I'd like to *not* be a walking, talking science experiment, thank you very much.

Plus, topically applied products go straight to your bloodstream, whereas ingested chemicals are filtered by the liver and kidneys. You also inhale these chemicals (especially with scented products) and eat them (as with lip and oral care products).

Now, you may be scratching your head and wondering, "How is this even possible?" And that is an absolutely fantastic question. Some countries have taken strict action to reduce the threat of these chemicals—the European Union has banned or restricted over 1,400 harmful chemicals from being used in skincare and cosmetics, and Canada has banned over 500. But in contrast, the United States has banned or restricted just 30 (at the time this book was published).

For decades, the beauty industry has been almost completely unregulated in the United States. Although the U.S. Food and Drug Administration (FDA) is charged with overseeing cosmetics, fragrance, and personal care products, its regulatory oversight is very limited.

- No product or ingredient requires FDA approval before going to market (with the sole exception being color additives).

- No product or ingredient requires safety testing. The FDA only "advises" manufacturers to test products and ingredients for safety before putting them on the market.

- The FDA cannot recall an unsafe product in the same way it can unsafe food. Although it can "request" that a product be recalled, the company selling the product must voluntarily issue the recall.

However, there has recently been some major progress in chemical safety regulation. Like the beauty industry, the chemical industry that produces many of the ingredients that go into cosmetic, fragrance and personal care products has also been largely unregulated thanks to major loopholes in the Toxic Substances Control Act. And so a number of politicians, consumer safety organizations and nonprofits working to protect public health and the environment have fought hard for stricter chemical safety regulations. Finally, in June 2016, a new law was passed to help close the loopholes. The Frank R. Lautenberg Chemical Safety for the 21st Century Act now mandates safety reviews for chemicals in active commerce, requires a safety finding for new chemicals before they can enter the market and makes information about chemicals more accessible to the public. These seem like no-brainers, right? It's certainly about time. And in the months after the Lautenberg Act was passed, the number of chemicals banned for use in cosmetics jumped from just a dozen to 30, showing promise for a less toxic future.

But even with this encouraging new chemical safety reform, it's important for consumers to be educated on this public health issue so they can make safer choices. The bottom line is that the beauty industry still isn't as tightly regulated as it should be, and we need to take protection into our own hands.

A number of commonly used skincare ingredients have been linked to some pretty serious health and skin issues.

It's good to get acquainted with these rabble-rousers so you can be on the lookout for them in product ingredient lists.

PARABENS: It is estimated that this family of preservatives is used in around 80 percent of all skincare products on the market. So, it's very likely that you have a product or two (or twenty-eight!) with at least one paraben in it. Members include propylparaben, methylparaben, butylparaben, isobutylparaben and ethylparaben, among others. Many of them have estrogen-mimicking properties and are known endocrine disruptors (i.e., they mess with your hormones). They have also been found in biopsy samples of breast tumors, which shows that they certainly penetrate the skin and make themselves at home in the body.

FRAGRANCE: This term is a catchall for any number of mysterious chemicals used to scent a product. Since it represents a grab bag of unnamed chemicals, this ingredient is especially troubling. Fragrance can irritate the skin, causing contact dermatitis. It is also a potential endocrine disruptor, known to irritate allergies and cause headaches, nausea and dizziness—I'm sure we've all had the unfortunate opportunity of being in an elevator or car with someone wearing far too much perfume or cologne and can attest to this!

SODIUM LAURYL SULFATE (SLS)/SODIUM LAURETH SULFATE (SLES): These surfactants are used in most conventional soaps and washes. They are known to be skin, lung and eye irritants. More concerning, SLS and SLES are often contaminated with ethylene oxide and its by-product 1,4-dioxane, both known carcinogens.

POLYETHYLENE GLYCOL (PEG): Like SLS/SLES, this penetration enhancer can be contaminated with two known carcinogens, ethylene oxide and 1,4-dioxane.

PROPYLENE GLYCOL: Oddly, this common skincare ingredient is also found in antifreeze, brake and hydraulic fluid, floor wax and paints. In skincare, it is used as a penetration enhancer, humectant, stabilizer and emulsifier. It has been known to cause breakouts and skin irritations, and there is concern that it may be contaminated with carcinogenic 1,4-dioxane, lead and/or arsenic.

DIETHANOLAMINE (DEA): This ingredient is most often used as an emulsifier or to adjust the pH of a product. In addition to being linked to odd skin growths, there is concern that DEA can form with other chemicals (either while in the bottle or in our bodies) to form nitrosamines, a number of which are known carcinogens.

TRICLOSAN: The U.S. Environmental Protection Agency (EPA) classifies this preservative and antibacterial agent as a probable human carcinogen. It is a known endocrine disruptor that affects the thyroid and reproductive systems. When mixed with chlorine—which is often found in tap water as a water treatment by-product—it can create dioxins and chloroform, two known carcinogens. This chemical is also known to bioaccumulate and has been found in breast milk.

TALC: This powder has a chemical composition similar to that of asbestos. It has been linked to ovarian cancer and respiratory issues. For this reason, thousands of women have filed lawsuits against Johnson & Johnson, claiming the firm's talc-containing baby powder caused their ovarian cancers. In a number of cases, the company has been found guilty of "negligent conduct" in the making and marketing of this product.

PETROLATUM (INCLUDING MINERAL OIL): This common emollient is a by-product of crude oil, making it an extremely cheap filler ingredient. It is commonly contaminated with 1,4-dioxane and coal tar, two known carcinogens. (To think that I used to use pure petroleum jelly as a lip balm!) It also creates a barrier on the skin, preventing oxygen from reaching the skin and sebum from escaping the pores. For this reason, it can cause blemishes.

OXYBENZONE: This common sunscreen is linked to allergies, hormone disruption, cellular damage and low birth weight. What makes it even scarier: It bioaccumulates in fat cells. Scarier still: Oxybenzone is known to kill coral reefs, which are home to 25 percent of all ocean life. For this reason, coral reefs are disappearing twice as fast as rain forests!

These chemicals aren't just found in skincare products. They're also commonly used in makeup and other personal care products.

THESE CHEMICALS ARE NOT ONLY A SOURCE OF PERSONAL POLLUTION, BUT OF ENVIRONMENTAL POLLUTION, TOO.

Chances are, if you care about your health you also care about the environment. And if you don't, you really ought to. Because our personal health and the health of the environment are intimately connected. Think about it: How can we be truly healthy if we're living in a toxic, polluted environment? We just can't! This is why I believe we should all do our part—no matter how small or seemingly insignificant—to care for this amazing planet we call home.

Making the switch to natural, nontoxic beauty and skincare products is one such way to do our part. Many ingredients found in beauty and skincare products are not biodegradable and don't break down. So, when they go down the drain (either when we're using them in the shower or washing them off), they end up in our waterways. Here, they alter the natural environment and negatively impact aquatic life.

Luckily, beauty doesn't have to come at such a cost: Safer skincare options exist!

As consumer awareness of this important issue increases, more and more companies are creating effective skincare and beauty products without all of the hazardous ingredients. In fact, the market is booming! This means that natural, nontoxic products aren't just available online and at health stores anymore, but have even made their way into big chain stores.

One of the simplest ways to spot safer skincare options is by the seal(s) they may be carrying on their labels.

 USDA ORGANIC/NATIONAL ORGANIC PROGRAM (NOP). Product must contain all or mostly agricultural ingredients, and can meet the USDA/NOP organic production, handling, processing and labeling standards.

 THE SOIL ASSOCIATION. At least 95 percent of product ingredients must be organic. If an ingredient is available organically, it must be used. All nonorganic ingredients must meet strict health and environmental standards.

CCOF (CALIFORNIA CERTIFIED ORGANIC FARMERS) CERTIFIED ORGANIC. At least 70 percent of all ingredients are organic.

 ECOCERT ORGANIC COSMETIC. At least 95 percent of all plant-based ingredients in the formula and at least 10 percent of all ingredients by weight must be organic.

 ECOCERT NATURAL COSMETIC. At least 50 percent of all plant-based ingredients in the formula at least 5 percent of all ingredients by weight must be organic.

When you see these specific labels on products, you can be sure that these products are being kept to the standards set out by the certification requirements.

That being said, a product does not necessarily have be certified organic or bear one of these seals to be a safe, nontoxic product. It can be an expensive and time-consuming process for small beauty and skincare companies to get these seals on their products, and some just don't see the necessity.

The absolute best way to know whether a product is safe is by carefully checking the ingredient label. Of course, reading ingredient labels feels like reading a foreign language you certainly did *not* study in high school! Fortunately, there are a few of helpful resources available to help you translate.

THE ENVIRONMENTAL WORKING GROUP'S SKIN DEEP® DATABASE. You can easily search individual ingredients as well as products for safety using this website. Each is given a ranking from zero to ten, zero being completely safe and ten being toxic sludge in a jar. You can also use the site to find safer alternatives.

THE ENVIRONMENTAL WORKING GROUP'S HEALTHY LIVING PHONE APP. This app allows you to scan product (food and home cleaning in addition to skincare and beauty) barcodes, quickly pulling up safety data. It's a great tool to have when out shopping.

THE THINK DIRTY PHONE® APP. Similar to the Environmental Working Group's Healthy Living phone app, this app features a barcode scanner for quick results. I've found that its data varies slightly from the Healthy Living app, so I use both to get the most comprehensive product information possible.

The idea of tossing all of your skincare products in the trash and finding natural alternatives can be overwhelming, so start slow with just one or two products. Although I mostly focus on facial skincare in this book, I suggest beginning your transition to natural skincare by switching out your body wash and lotion for safer alternatives, since these products are applied to the greatest area of skin. (Plus, a natural oil such as coconut, grapeseed or apricot kernel oil makes for an amazing, all-natural, single-ingredient body moisturizer!)

CAUTION: BEWARE OF GREENWASHING!

Marketing professionals sometimes exploit the increased demand for healthier, natural products in product branding and advertising. They use vague buzzwords that are not regulated and can be used at will regardless of a product's ingredients—such words as *natural* and *organic* (yep!), or *eco*, *pure*, *botanical* and *mineral*. So, a product "naturally created with the organic essence of nature's botanicals" may sound super-duper crunchy and clean when in fact it may very well be chock-full of unnatural, toxic garbage. Another common greenwashing tactic is to draw attention to certain ingredients that a product does not contain. For example, a product may be paraben-free or SLS-free, but it may also contain other unhealthy ingredients.

So, the onus is on consumers to be educated and choose wisely! Greenwashers want to razzle-dazzle us with pretty pictures of flowers and nice-sounding words. Ignore these. Turn over whatever it is you're looking at and carefully inspect that ingredient label, because this is where the truth lies. What do you see? A bunch of chemical-sounding terms? Any member of the paraben family? The ever mysterious "fragrance"? If yes, put that baby right back on the shelf.

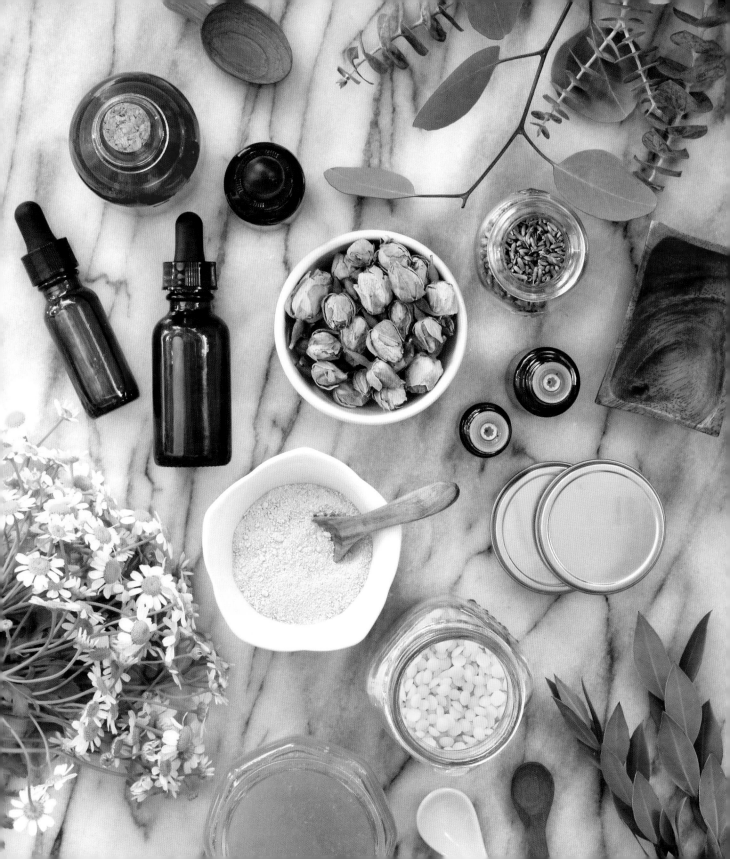

Making your own skincare products is a great way to know exactly what you're putting on your skin.

After all, you are the one putting all of the ingredients into the product!

The world of DIY skincare and beauty has been blowing up recently as more and more people learn about the dangers of conventional products. Also because it is just so darn fun and easy to create decadent products with your own two hands! *An organic exfoliating enzyme facemask that I can make with ingredients from my pantry? Yes, please!*

And yes, these incredibly simple ingredients that you use to make your products are extremely beneficial for the skin. Mother Nature has provided us with an amazing abundance of therapeutic herbs, flowers, clays, butters and oils that the skin absolutely adores—they provide skin with hydrating lipids, protective antioxidants, critical vitamins and minerals and so much more.

There are a seemingly endless number of ingredients to use in homemade skincare formulations. In this book, we will look at just a few of the basics as we scratch at the surface of DIY skincare.

DIY NATURAL SKINCARE BASICS

BUTTERS: You can think of butters as superthick lotion. They're solid fats that moisturize skin with nourishing lipids and are filled with vitamins, including the protective antioxidants vitamins A, C and E.

- Shea butter
- Cocoa butter
- Kokum butter
- Mango butter

OILS: Like dietary oils, skincare oils are essentially liquid fats. Similar to butters, they moisturize and nourish skin while providing crucial vitamins and protective antioxidants.

- Blemish-prone skin
  - Grapeseed oil
  - Hemp seed oil
  - Pumpkin seed oil
  - Tamanu oil
- Aging/mature skin
  - Apricot kernel oil
  - Argan oil
  - Rosehip oil

- Oily skin
  - Grapeseed oil
  - Jojoba oil
  - Rosehip oil
- Dry skin
  - Apricot kernel oil
  - Avocado oil
  - Sweet almond oil
- Irritated/sensitive skin
  - Apricot kernel oil

ESSENTIAL OILS: These concentrated plant extracts are extremely potent. They provide unique benefits to the skin ranging from reducing inflammation to improving cellular turnover, and they can also be used to help preserve (to an extent) homemade skincare products. These are some of my favorite skin-loving essential oils: carrot seed, frankincense, geranium, lavender, rose, rosemary and tea tree.

HERBS: Just as herbs provide the body with anti-inflammatory and antioxidant benefits when consumed, they provide the skin with similar benefits. They are sometimes applied directly to the skin but can also be infused in oils or liquids, which are then applied to the skin. These are some of my favorite herbs for the skin: calendula, chamomile, lavender and tumeric.

CLAYS: Packed with important minerals, clays help draw impurities and oil from the skin. These are a few of my favorite clays: bentonite clay, French green clay and kaolin clay.

VEGETABLE GLYCERIN: This natural humectant draws water to the top layers of the skin and keeps it there.

WITCH HAZEL EXTRACT: This natural toner has anti-inflammatory and astringent properties. It also helps to maintain the skin's natural pH.

ALOE VERA: Extracted from the leaves of aloe plants, this gel is a natural humectant, pulling water to the skin. In addition to providing hydration, it's great at soothing irritated skin.

RAW HONEY: This sticky sweetness is a natural skincare staple! It's not only a natural humectant that helps to draw hydration to the skin, but it's also filled with antioxidants and helps fight bacteria.

Also, never discount other food ingredients! Apple cider vinegar, avocado, oats and baking soda are all staples in my natural skincare routine

Ready to kick unhealthy chemicals to the curb?

Once you know about the unhealthy ingredients in your skincare products, it's difficult to turn back to them. Luckily, you're now armed with the knowledge of how to find safer alternatives—including those you can make at home!

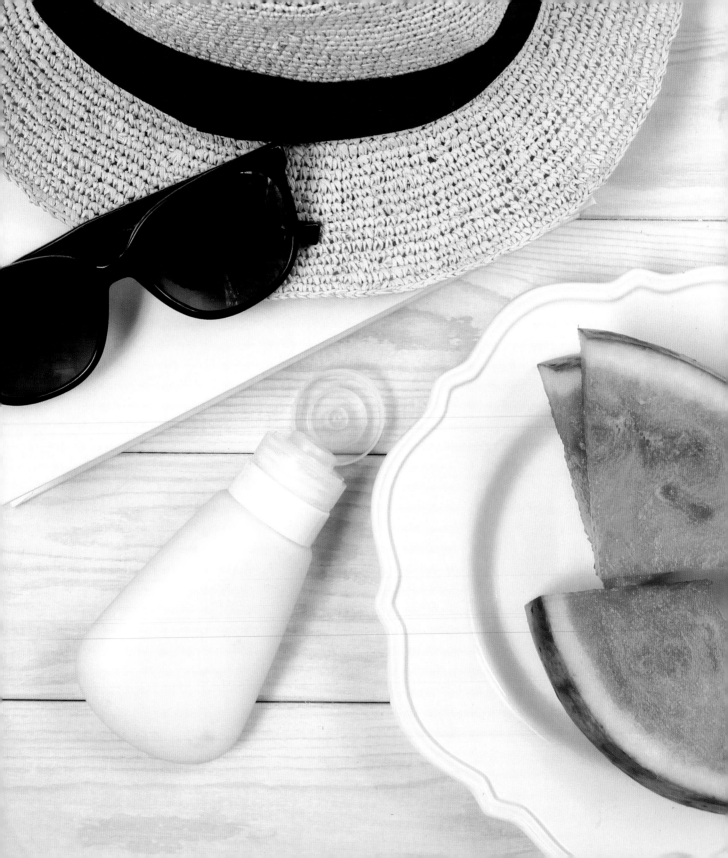

PREVENT FREE RADICAL DAMAGE
THE BEST OFFENSE IS A GOOD DEFENSE

Free radicals have a bad reputation and for a good reason.

We've already discussed these bad boys a bit, but here's the quick and dirty in case you need a little refresher: Free radicals are unstable molecules that can cause inflammation, destroy collagen, damage DNA, impair the cellular structure and oxidize sebum (which increases the risk of blemishes). And while free radicals are a natural result of the body's metabolism as well as a cause and a result of inflammation, the skin is uniquely exposed to a greater amount of free radicals from external sources.

The most significant external source of free radical damage to the skin: the sun. The sun's UV rays have been shown to accelerate skin aging (called photoaging) and damage DNA, which can lead to skin cancer. For this reason, we're bombarded with messages to slather on sunscreen at all times. But this is a very tricky topic since our bodies require adequate sun exposure for vitamin D production. "The sunshine vitamin" is absolutely critical for good health and the prevention of all cancers (yes, even skin cancer). In fact, some argue that our current epidemic of vitamin D deficiency is occurring because we've all been "scared sunless" due to increased rates of skin cancer, and that this may actually be far more detrimental to our health than sun exposure itself. It's a heavily debated, pretty sticky situation, and one in which we need to safely strike a delicate balance between adequate sun exposure and the prevention of UV damage.

Environmental pollutants are also a significant source of free radical damage. Automobile exhaust, power plants, factories, industrial sites, construction sites and fires are all sources of microscopic air pollutants. These nanoparticles are extremely small—some are twenty times smaller than our pores. This means that they don't just sit on the skin waiting patiently for us to wash them off. Oh, no. Instead, their small size allows them to penetrate deep into the skin's layers, sometimes even making it to the bloodstream.

Fortunately, there are some relatively simple steps we can take to prevent free radical damage.

When it comes to preventing free radical damage, it's a matter of:

1. Practicing safe sun exposure

2. Protecting the skin from environmental pollutants

3. Using topical antioxidants to neutralize free radicals

Practicing safe sun exposure is critical for protecting the skin from free radical-generating UV rays.

However, safe sun exposure does not mean avoiding the daylight like a vampire or slathering your skin in sunscreen each time you step outside. It's about getting enough exposure for the skin to synthesize vitamin D without experiencing any damage. With safe sun exposure, the skin should not burn, but gradually (over days and weeks) turn slightly tan. Because while overexposure to the sun most certainly causes photoaging and DNA damage, safe sun exposure provides the body and skin with the vitamin D it needs to protect itself from such damage and so much more.

Of course, anyone who has ever been caught in the sun without protection knows that it doesn't take too long for the skin to begin burning. So, safe sun exposure includes shade, protective clothing, hats and sunscreen. I personally wear sunblock on my face every day to prevent photoaging and apply sunblock to my body when I know I will be in direct sunlight for extended periods of time, such as while at the beach, during a backyard barbecue or on an extended hike.

When using sunscreen, it's important to be discerning so that we don't put ourselves at further risk for UV damage or skin cancer. Many people simply look at the sun protection factor (SPF) value when it comes to sunscreen, but many sunscreens—even those with SPF 100—don't provide adequate protection from UVA rays, which penetrate the skin more deeply than UVB rays and are the primary culprit in skin aging and cancer. When it comes to topical sun protection, natural mineral sunblocks are the best option, since they offer immediate, long-lasting, broad-spectrum protection (that is, they protect skin from both UVB and UVA rays). Plus, mineral sunblocks won't add to your body burden. Because remember how your skin is your body's largest organ and the majority of what you apply to it gets absorbed directly into the bloodstream? Well, chemical sunscreen depends on this—it works by the active ingredients absorbing into the skin where they then absorb the sun's rays. But some of these active ingredients (such as homosalate and oxybenzone) have been linked to endocrine disruption, organ system toxicity or developmental and reproductive toxicity. They are not exactly ingredients you want to be slathering all over your body! When you choose a mineral sunblock made with non-nano active ingredients, however, the active ingredient does not absorb into the skin. Instead it acts as a protective layer on top of your skin, reflecting rays like a mirror. Mineral sunscreen is also less irritating to sensitive skin. While some of the active ingredients used in chemical sunscreens trigger allergies and skin reactions, mineral sunscreen rarely causes such irritation. In fact, zinc oxide—one of the most popular mineral sunscreen ingredients—is actually used in natural diaper rash creams to soothe irritated little bottoms.

Take a close look at the ingredients list—not just active ingredients! You will still find some mineral sunscreens with unhealthy ingredients, such as endocrine-disrupting artificial fragrance and retinyl palmitate, which is believed to increase the rate at which cancerous cells divide when combined with sunlight (not a good thing, considering you use sunscreen when you're exposed to sunlight).

It's also important to protect your skin from environmental pollutants.

Unless you want to live in a bubble, it's unfortunately impossible to avoid air pollution. However, there are certain measures you can take to protect the skin from its damaging effects. The good news: They're incredibly simple and likely measures you already take without knowing this added benefit!

Since environmental pollutants settle on the skin throughout the day, it's important to wash your face every evening. Occasional exfoliation can also help to get rid of any environmental pollutants that may have settled into the top layers of the skin.

Applying moisturizer also helps to create a barrier on the skin, preventing environmental pollutants from penetrating the skin's layers. Instead, they cling to the moisturizer like bugs to a windshield, waiting for you to wash them away.

Certain skincare ingredients also play a key role in neutralizing free radicals.

Some of the very same antioxidants that work wonders for the skin from the inside out can have the same effect when applied topically. Vitamins A, C and E, as well as the antioxidants found in green tea, cacao and berries, can all help to neutralize free radicals when applied to the skin. For this reason, most natural skincare products contain certain oils and butters naturally rich in the antioxidant vitamins or extracts of antioxidant-rich foods. The Antioxidant Green Tea Toner (page 154) and Protecting Matcha Mask (page 166) both help neutralize free radicals topically by imparting the amazing antioxidant properties of green tea onto the skin.

Taking these steps to prevent and neutralize free radical exposure is key to maintaining healthy skin.

Free radicals don't just accelerate skin aging and increase the risk of blemishes—they cause DNA damage that can develop into cancer. Fortunately, as we've just learned, we can quite easily and effectively take precautionary steps to prevent free radicals from doing their dirty work on our skin!

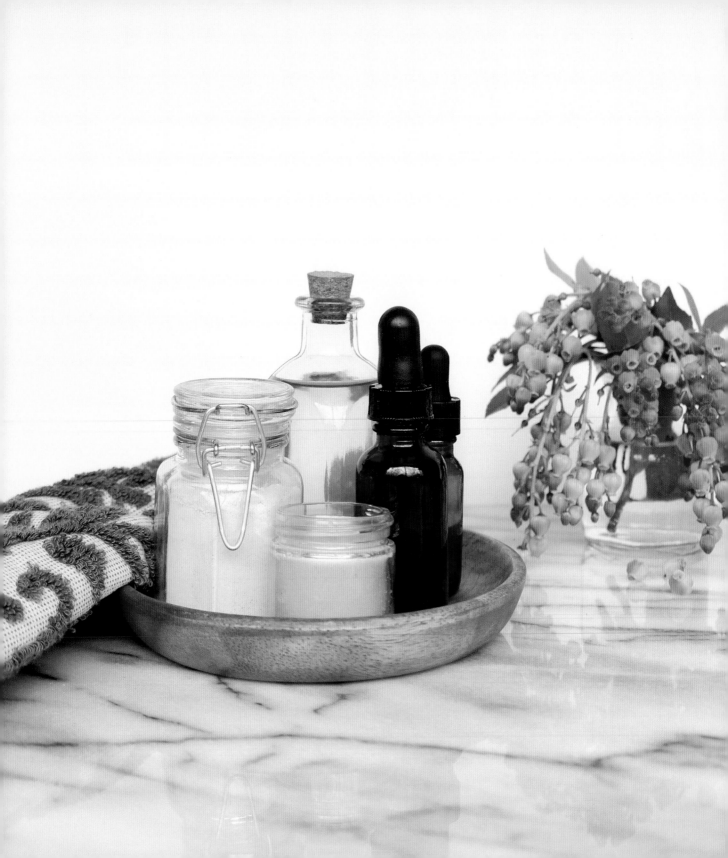

SIMPLIFY YOUR SKINCARE ROUTINE

JUST 3 STEPS: CLEANSE, PERFECT, PROTECT

Reflection time: Are you fighting against your skin?

Washing your face three, four or five times a day? Using astringents upon masks upon scrubs upon peels?

That used to be me. And though my intentions were good, I was doing more harm than good to my poor, inflamed skin.

Harsh and excessive skincare can strip the skin of its protective oils and throw its pH off balance. When this happens, the skin becomes dry and irritated, and often tries to bring itself back into equilibrium by producing excess oil, increasing the risk for breakouts. An altered pH also allows the bad bacteria living on the skin—including the dreaded *P. acnes* bacteria—to grow and thrive.

It's important to work with your skin and not against it. Simple is the best way to go when it comes to a skincare routine because the skin really doesn't require too much—a daily cleanse, the occasional toner, mask or scrub to help perfect tone and texture, and a nourishing moisturizer rich in vitamins and antioxidants.

When it comes to simplifying your skincare routine, it's a matter of:

1. Cleansing your skin appropriately

2. Perfecting your complexion with pH balancing toners, gentle exfoliation and the occasional mask

3. Protecting your skin with a nourishing moisturizer

To soap or not to soap? That is the question.

Chances are, if you're not doing anything else to your skin, you're washing it. And although cleansers get more playtime going down the drain than they do actually on our face, they can still significantly impact our complexion.

There are a couple of good reasons to avoid using soap on the face. Soap can dry the skin by stripping it of its natural oils. More important, soap has an alkaline pH of around 9, whereas the pH of skin is naturally slightly acidic at around 5.5. The alkaline pH of soap can disrupt the skin's pH, causing irritation and interfering with the skin-shedding process. This is an especially important issue for those with sensitive, dry or blemish-prone skin. But I'm going to tell you something: I'm a soap fan! I'm sure many, many skincare experts would grunt at this declaration in disgust, but it's what works best for my skin. If you also prefer some suds, it's important to find or make a mild soap that does the job without doing it too well (i.e., totally stripping the skin). A natural, oil-based bar soap made of coconut or olive oil and little else is a good way to go. The recipe for my personal favorite face wash—Nourishing Honey Face Wash—can be found on page 145. And we'll discuss the important role a good toner can play in rebalancing skin pH in just a bit.

A good moisturizer is key to maintaining glowing skin.

THERE ARE JUST SO MANY REASONS TO MOISTURIZE

- Moisturized skin feels soft and looks smooth.

- Moisturized skin heals more quickly than dry skin.

- Moisturized skin appears more plump and youthful.

- Moisturizer creates a barrier on your skin, protecting it from age-accelerating environmental pollutants.

A good moisturizer will also provide your skin with vitamins, minerals, antioxidants and other beneficial ingredients it needs to help banish blemishes, soothe irritated skin and slow the signs of aging. But finding a good moisturizer is no easy feat! Not only do we need to find one that does everything just mentioned, but that also doesn't clog pores, make us look like a shiny mess and is nontoxic.

You'll recall from our conversation about dry skin, way back on page 21, that skin "moisture" really has to do with two things, hydration and moisture. Hydration is related to water while moisture is related to oil. When the skin is untouched and no skincare products are involved, skin hydration is totally dependent on body hydration (i.e., how much water you have had to drink) and skin moisture is provided by the skin's own sebum, which locks in hydration and prevents it from evaporating. A good moisturizer mimics this natural relationship.

Although water is a common ingredient in skincare products, it really doesn't do much to hydrate the skin. In fact, it can cause the skin to become even drier as it evaporates, taking some of the water content of the skin along with it. Humectants, on the other hand, provide amazing hydration—they have the superpower to actually draw water from the environment and pull it into your skin. I know, it sounds a little bizarre and totally impossible. But they're very real and work wonders. Aloe, hyaluronic acid and vegetable glycerin are natural humectants commonly used in moisturizers.

Just as the skin's natural sebum keeps hydration in the skin by preventing it from evaporating, so do oils and butters. It's no secret that my personal favorite moisturizer is oil. As with the Oil Cleansing Method, oil used as a moisturizer actually helps keep pores clear by the principle of like-dissolves-like. Plus, applying oil to your skin can actually trick your sebaceous glands to produce less oil. Oils are also naturally rich with antioxidants, vitamins and fatty acids, all of which your skin depends on to maintain its glow. See why I love them so?

Although oil and butters alone make for wonderful moisturizers, if you'd like the added benefit of hydration, be sure to look for natural humectants on the ingredient label of potential moisturizers. And of course, you can always make your own! The Ultramoisturizing Lotion (page 173) combines oils and humectants for a ridiculously soft complexion. But if you are an oil fan such as myself, you can still treat your skin to the hydrating powers of humectants by spritzing the Hydrating Rose Facial Mist (page 174) before applying your oil.

SKINCARE ISN'T JUST ABOUT THE PRODUCTS YOU APPLY TO YOUR SKIN—IT'S ABOUT HOW YOU INTERACT WITH IT, TOO.

Remember to keep your hands and hair away from your face! This is especially important if you struggle with acne, since you can easily transfer pore-clogging dirt and oil from your hands and hair to your face.

Be sure to also keep a close eye on your body and hair care products. These may contain ingredients that are irritating to your skin or clogging your pores.

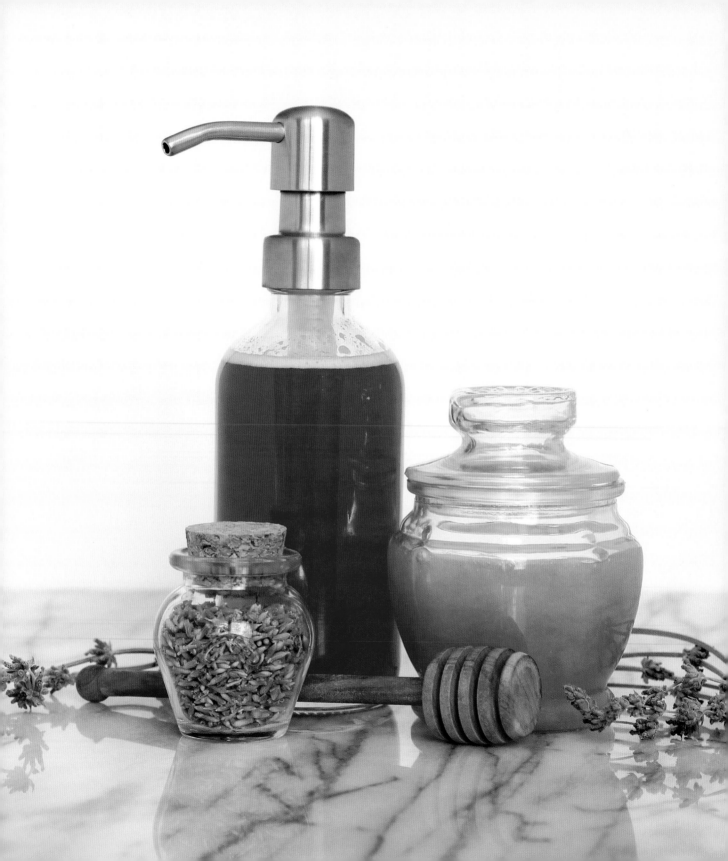

Natural DIY Skincare Recipes

• • •

HEY, THERE'S FOOD ON YOUR FACE

SKINCARE SO NATURAL, YOU COULD LITERALLY EAT IT

Warning: Making your own skincare products is extremely addictive.

Be prepared to fall down a rabbit hole of face oils, essential oils, clays, mason jars, small wooden spoons (okay, this one may just be my own strange fixation!) and dried herbs. You'll never look at seaweed or coffee beans the same way again, and you'll start wondering, "Should I make a mask with this?" every time you're in the produce section of the grocery store.

But unlike most other addictions, making your own skincare products is 100 percent healthy! Not only are you feeding your skin from the outside—neutralizing free radicals or fighting inflammation using Mother Nature's bounty—you're also protecting your body from the toxic ingredients found in conventional, store-bought skincare products. And in the long run, your bank account will thank you for making your own skincare products rather than turning to high-end beauty companies or the spa.

Do keep in mind that these products will have a shorter shelf life than store-bought skincare items.

Particular care should be taken to prevent bacteria growth. For this reason, many of the recipes have a small yield—it is better to make a facemask every week than to worry about mold growth. Also, very few of the recipes include water since water allows for bacteria growth.

That being said, aloe is naturally comprised of mostly water. Particular care should be taken to avoid bacteria growth in the recipes that call for aloe, and you will see that I have included certain essential oils in these recipes to help with this. I advise against using aloe vera gel collected from the plant for those recipes that have a larger yield, since aloe vera gel purchased at the store contains a small amount of natural preservative.

Products that are made of oils and butters will have a much longer shelf life. As long as moisture does not enter the product, the issue with these is not bacteria growth but rancidity. As we've discussed, fats and oils rancidify, some more quickly than others. Many face oils are comprised of delicate essential fatty acids. Although these are great for the skin when applied topically, they do go rancid within a few months.

BACTERIA HAVE NO PLACE IN YOUR HOMEMADE BEAUTY PRODUCTS!

To extend the life of your homemade skincare products and protect yourself, it is extremely important to take special care to prevent bacterial growth in the products.

- Use a clean work space.
- Wash your hands before starting.
- Sterilize your glass containers.
- Make sure your containers are completely dry before filling them.
- Keep moisture out of your products while both making and using them.

If you notice any sort of growth or change in scent or texture, don't chance it! Discard the product and make a new batch.

The recipes that follow are to help you get started, but feel free to get creative!

Do you prefer a particular oil, essential oil or butter? Go ahead and use it! Want to add some lavender to the Chamomile Rose Cleansing Grains (page 146)? Some cacao to the Moisturizing Avo-Nana Mask (page 169)? Why not!?

Nourishing Honey Face Wash

Honey has a long history of beauty and skincare use, going back all the way to the O.G. (Original Glamazon), Cleopatra. And it's no wonder—honey naturally fights bacteria while providing skin with a dose of antioxidants and locking in moisture as a natural humectant.

This face wash is a great way to give your skin a daily dose of honey and its glow-getting benefits. It's particularly great for those of us who prefer some suds. Castile soap is a wonderful natural soap that easily removes excess oil, pollutants and makeup. The nourishing honey perfectly balances the harshness of the castile soap, keeping skin from becoming stripped by drawing moisture to the skin as a natural humectant. Lavender works wonders for all skin types, also helping to keep bacteria and inflammation away.

YIELD: 8 OZ (240 ML)

¾ cup (180 ml) raw honey

¼ cup (60 ml) castile soap

20 drops lavender essential oil

10 drops tea tree essential oil

In a bottle, combine all the ingredients and shake vigorously to blend.

Gently rub a coin-size amount into wet skin.

*See photo on page 142.

NOTES

The ingredients may separate over time, so be sure to give the bottle a little shake every once in a while!

Since castile soap has a pH of around 9, you may wish to occasionally use a toner to rebalance the skin's pH and keep it from getting irritated. Check out the pH-Balancing Toner (page 150).

Chamomile Rose Cleansing Grains

These cleansing grains are a one-stop shop for all of your skin needs. They wash away impurities without the use of potentially irritating soap while providing a buff gentle enough to be had daily.

This particular recipe contains goodies that benefit all skin types. Oats may have a reputation for being boring but are actually quite the opposite—not only do they calm irritated skin, but they also contain natural saponins that absorb excess oil and cleanse the skin. Rose petals are rich in the antioxidant powerhouse vitamin C and act as a mild astringent, keeping pores clear and tight. Chamomile soothes irritated, inflamed skin. Last but certainly not least, French green clay absorbs dirt and excess oil while providing skin with a healthy dose of minerals.

YIELD: 4 OZ (115 G)

4 tbsp (22 g) oats

2 tbsp (4 g) loosely packed rose petals

2 tbsp (4 g) loosely packed chamomile flowers

3 tbsp (27 g) French green clay

In a high-speed blender, food processor or coffee grinder, grind the oats, rose petals and chamomile flowers together into a fine powder. Transfer the finely ground mixture to a jar, add the French green clay and give the mixture a shake to blend the ingredients.

To use, mix about 1 teaspoon (5 g) of cleansing grains with a small amount of water in the palm of your hand to form a thick paste. Rub the grains into your face using gentle, circular motions. Rinse and bask in the beauty of your skin!

NOTES

To avoid bacteria growth, make sure your hands are clean and dry before scooping the grains from the jar and to securely close the jar after you are finished.

Since these grains do very mildly exfoliate the skin, use them no more than once a day.

Cleansing grains are not fantastic at removing makeup, so be sure to remove makeup (a little bit of oil does the trick) before using.

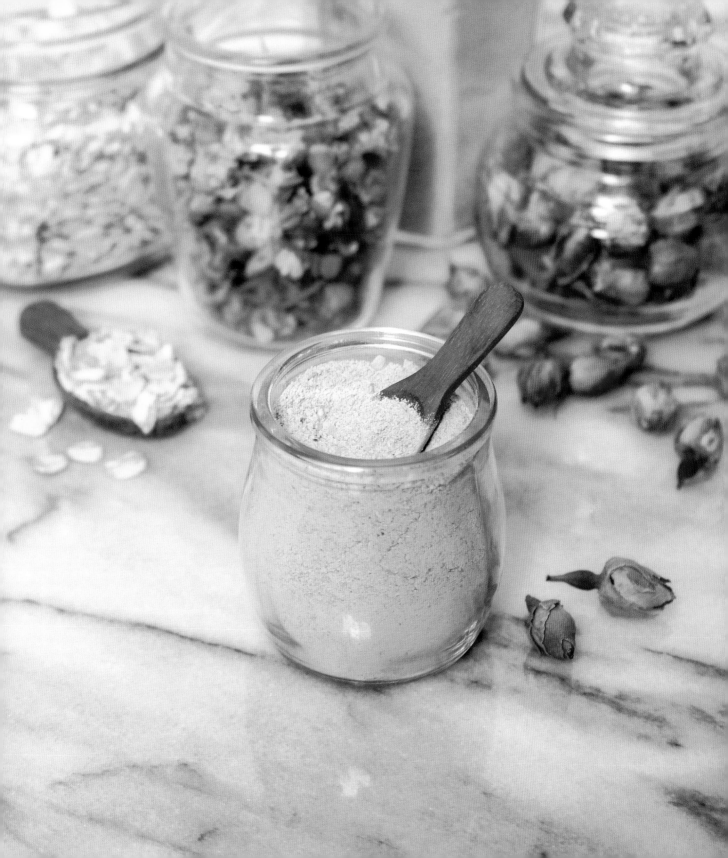

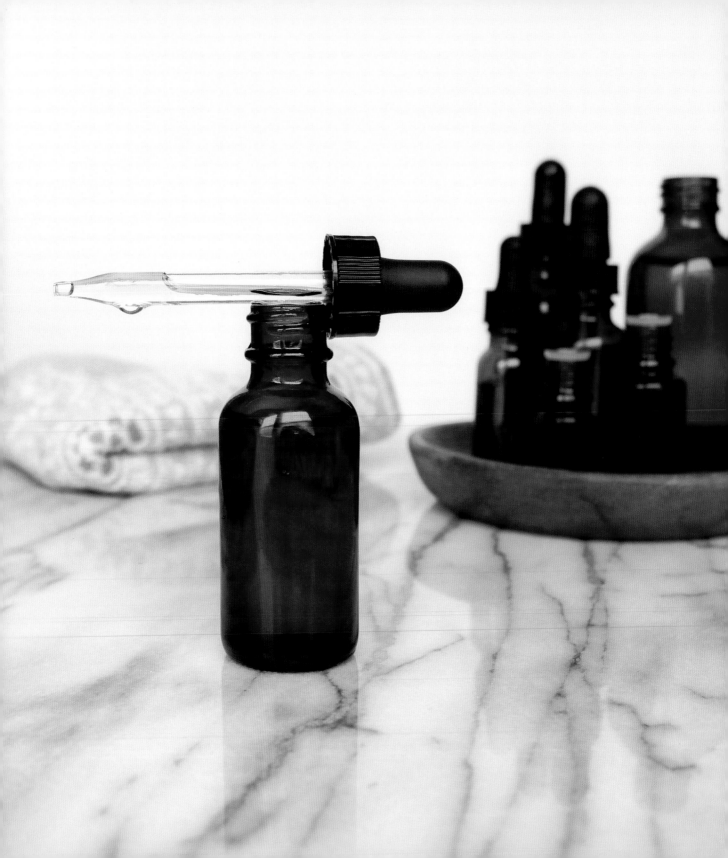

Like-Dissolves-Like Cleansing Oil

Hopefully by this point I've convinced you of the many magical wonders oils can do for the skin—not only are they filled with vitamins and antioxidants to protect and feed the skin from the outside, but they also help keep pores clear by the principle of like-dissolves-like. For this reason, oil is commonly used as a method of cleaning the skin, as we discussed in detail on page 138.

This basic cleansing oil is great for just starting out with the Oil Cleansing Method. Hazelnut oil is naturally astringent, making it the backbone of the recipe. Grapeseed oil is easily absorbed and beneficial for all skin concerns, from acne to aging. Avocado oil is richly moisturizing, balancing the other two oils, which are on the drier side. Lavender, rosemary and tea tree essential oil all help to keep skin clean.

YIELD: 4 OZ (120 ML)

4 tbsp (60 ml) grapeseed oil

2 tbsp (30 ml) hazelnut oil

2 tbsp (30 ml) avocado oil

15 drops lavender essential oil

10 drops rosemary essential oil

8 drops tea tree essential oil

In a 4-ounce (120-ml) dropper bottle, combine all the ingredients, put the cap on and give it a good shake to blend everything together.

To use, massage 10 or so drops into your entire face. Lay a hot damp towel on top of your face, then quickly lay a second dry washcloth on top to trap the moisture and heat. Let it sit for 1 to 2 minutes, or until the wet washcloth cools. Repeat, then gently wipe the water and excess oil from the skin with the dry washcloth at the end. (More details on the Oil Cleansing Method can be found on page 138.)

NOTES

If you have dry skin or find this mixture too drying, dilute it by adding more avocado oil. Reduce the amount of hazelnut oil in the next batch.

If you have oily or acne-prone skin, replace the avocado oil with grapeseed or pumpkin seed oil.

pH-Balancing Toner

Apple cider vinegar is the duct tape of the naturalista's medicine cabinet: It does just about everything! Including balancing the pH of the skin's acid mantle.

This toner is beneficial to all skin types, but especially oily and acne-prone skin. By bringing the skin's pH back into balance, it prevents irritation and closes the door to the acne-causing bacteria that thrive in more neutral conditions. The natural alpha hydroxy acids in apple cider vinegar also help to remove pore-clogging dead skin cells, tighten the appearance of pores and decrease the appearance of scars. Lavender essential oil helps to mask the scent of the vinegar as well as further improve skin's tone and texture.

YIELD: 2 OZ (60 ML)

1 tbsp (15 ml) apple cider vinegar

3 tbsp (45 ml) purified water

8 drops lavender essential oil

In a small glass bottle, combine all ingredients and shake to combine.

Shake gently before each use and apply with a cotton ball or clean washcloth. Follow with moisturizer.

NOTES

How often to use this toner depends on your unique skin, but you're likely to find that it's unnecessary to use it every day. I suggest using it every other day, seeing how your skin fares and going from there.

This toner is especially great for those with acne or oily skin. Those with dry skin may find it further dries their skin, potentially causing irritation.

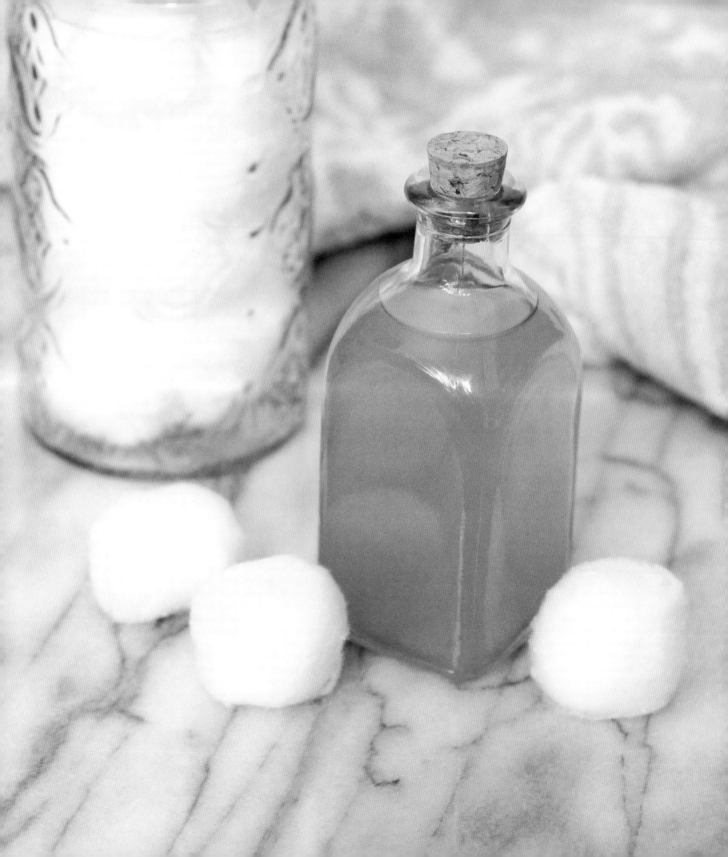

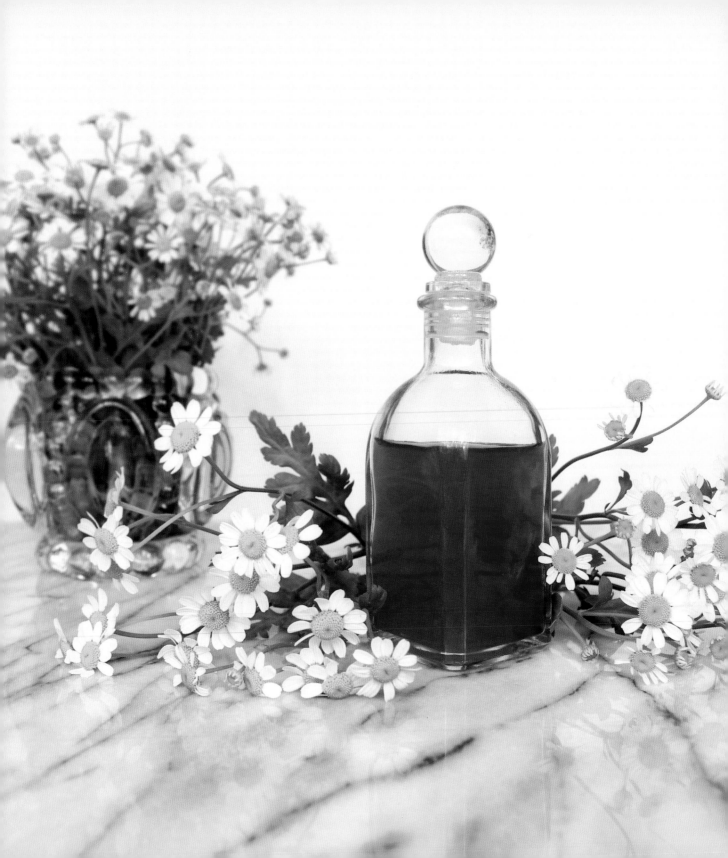

Calming Chamomile Aloe Face Toner

When I was younger, chamomile tea was my mother's antidote for all my stresses. She'd sit me down at the kitchen table and have me tell her my troubles (you know, so-and-so was mean to me or so-and-so didn't like me back) while I drank the tea. With each sip, I felt a little calmer. Okay, yes, venting is undoubtedly cathartic, but the tea played an important role, too—chamomile is an herb that has been used for centuries to relieve muscle tension and promote relaxation.

Chamomile has similar benefits for stressed-out skin. When applied topically, it fights inflammation and calms irritated skin. Witch hazel and aloe are also well-known skin-soothers, further helping to reduce irritation. To boot, witch hazel helps fight bacteria, balance the skin's pH and tighten the appearance of pores while aloe provides skin with a wash of moisture.

YIELD: 3 OZ (90 ML)

2 tsp (1 g) dried chamomile

4 tbsp (60 ml) witch hazel extract

2 tbsp (30 ml) aloe vera gel

Place the dried chamomile in a jar and pour the witch hazel on top. Screw the lid onto the jar and give the jar a little swirl to saturate the flowers. Let the mixture steep for at least 8 hours.

After allowing the mixture adequate time to steep, strain the flowers from the infused witch hazel, using cheesecloth or a coffee filter, giving them a squeeze to remove as much witch hazel as possible.

Pour the chamomile-infused witch hazel into a bottle or jar, add the aloe vera gel and stir.

Apply to clean skin, using a cotton ball or clean washcloth, and follow with moisturizer.

NOTES

Be sure to look for as natural an aloe vera gel as you can find. No, aloe is not bright green in real life! The bottle should indicate that it contains more than 99 percent natural aloe (with the remaining less than 1 percent of ingredients being natural preservatives).

Instead of using loose dried chamomile, alternatively you can use 1 chamomile tea bag. Simply cut the bag open and empty the tea into the witch hazel to infuse.

Antioxidant Green Tea Toner

This Antioxidant Green Tea Toner is incredibly simple because it just doesn't need to be any more complicated. The antioxidant powers of green tea combined with the natural toning properties of witch hazel provide skin with the ultimate protection. This toner helps defend skin cells from damaging free radicals and protects sebum from blemish-provoking oxidation, all while maintaining the skin's delicate pH. It's therefore a great addition to anti-aging and anti-acne skincare routines alike, and it's especially perfect for adults with acne who are concerned about both issues simultaneously.

YIELD: 4 OZ (120 ML)

1 tbsp (3.5 g) loose green tea leaves

½ cup (120 ml) witch hazel extract

Place the green tea leaves in a jar and pour the witch hazel on top. Screw the lid onto the jar and give the jar a little swirl to saturate the tea. Let the mixture steep for at least 8 hours.

After allowing the mixture adequate time to steep, strain the tea from the infused witch hazel, using cheesecloth or a coffee filter, giving them a squeeze to remove as much witch hazel as possible.

Pour the infused witch hazel into a bottle or jar.

Apply to clean skin, using a cotton ball or clean cloth, and follow with moisturizer.

NOTE: Instead of using loose green tea leaves, alternatively you can use 2 green tea bags. Simply cut the bags open and empty the tea into the witch hazel to infuse.

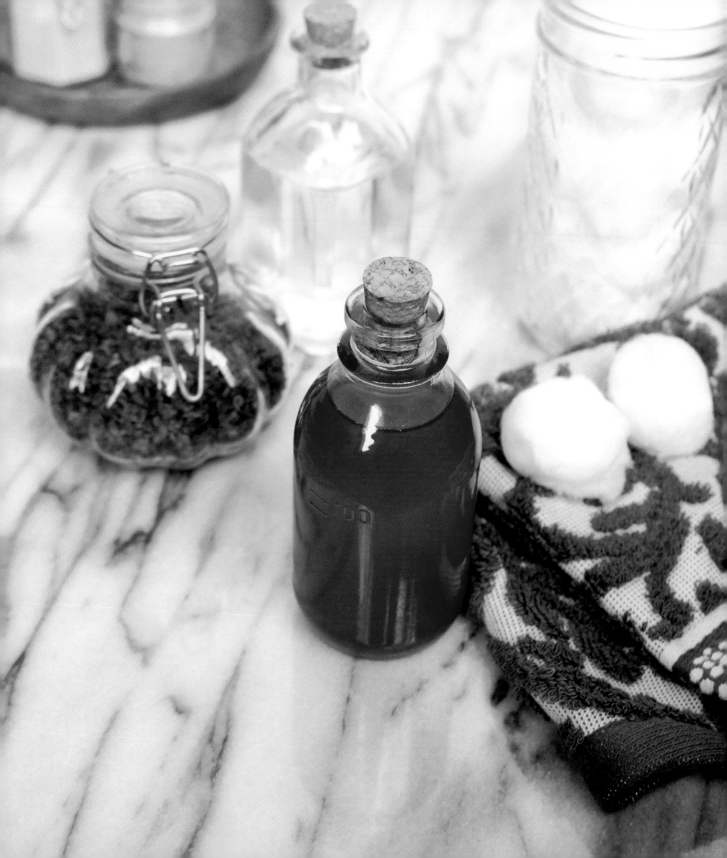

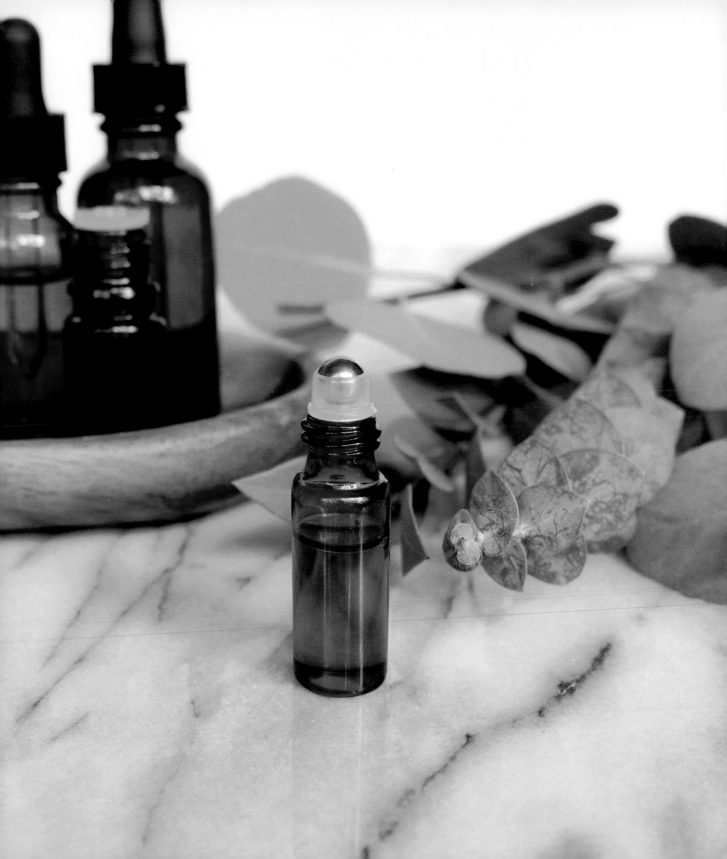

Blemish-Banishing Spot Treatment

When a zit rears its ugly head, you need to be ready to attack! And I don't mean with those itching fingers—picking at your skin often just makes things worse, aggravating inflammation, potentially spreading bacteria and increasing the risk of scarring.

This spot treatment contains ingredients that soothe inflamed skin as well as ward off bacteria, providing your skin with everything it needs to banish blemishes fast.

YIELD: 1 OZ (30 ML)

1 tbsp (15 ml) grapeseed oil

2 tsp (10 ml) tamanu oil

1 tsp (5 ml) tea tree oil

2 drops rosemary essential oil

In a 1-ounce (30-ml) glass dropper or roller bottle, combine everything and shake well.

Apply one drop directly to blemishes.

NOTE: Do not use tamanu oil if you are allergic to tree nuts. Use more grapeseed oil or pumpkin seed oil instead.

Shockingly Simple At-Home Microdermabrasion

"Did you treat yourself to a spa day?" they'll ask. When really, you simply tapped into the powers of the most multipurpose DIY agent out there: baking soda! Yep, this kitchen staple is a natural skincare must-have. And for just pennies, it mimics a $300 spa treatment like a pro.

Baking soda's extremely fine grain makes it an amazing exfoliant for delicate facial skin. As such, it helps to keep pores clear and stimulate collagen production. Aloe and vegetable glycerin provide moisture, protecting the delicate underlayer of skin that is now exposed. The result is smoother, brighter, spa-worthy skin.

YIELD: 1 USE

2 tsp (14 g) baking soda

½ tsp aloe vera gel

¼ tsp vegetable glycerin

In a small bowl, simply mix all the ingredients together into a smooth paste.

Massage into damp, clean skin using gentle, circular motions.

Wash off with warm water and follow with moisturizer.

NOTES

Baking soda has an alkaline pH and so can neutralize the skin's naturally acidic pH, potentially causing irritation. If you notice any irritation, you can bring your skin's pH back into balance with the pH-Balancing Toner (page 150).

To avoid irritating the skin, do not to use this treatment more than once a week.

Be sure to look for as natural an aloe vera gel as you can find (hint: aloe is not naturally green). The bottle should indicate that it contains more than 99 percent natural aloe (with the remaining less than 1 percent of ingredients being natural preservatives).

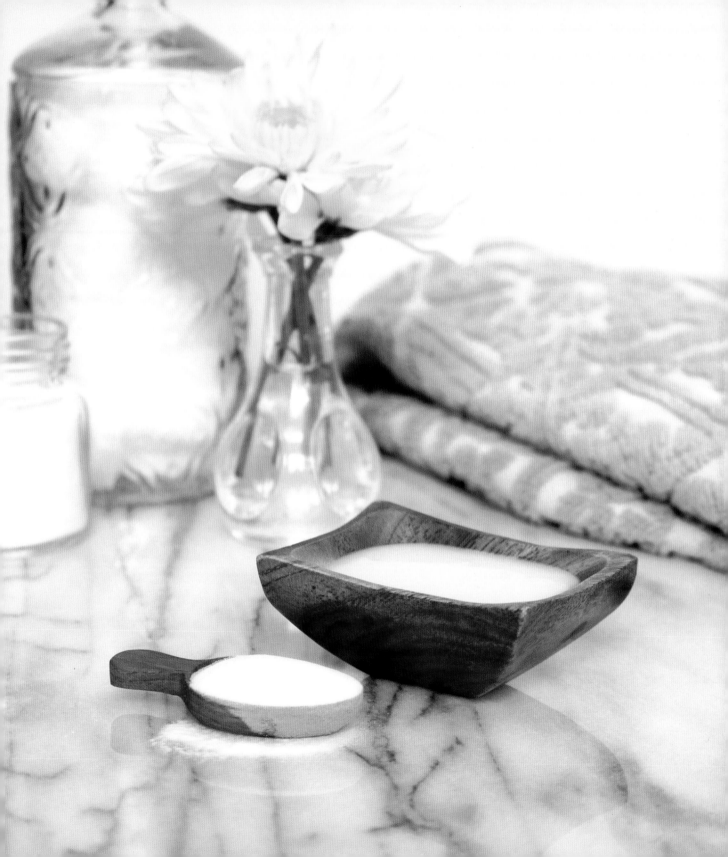

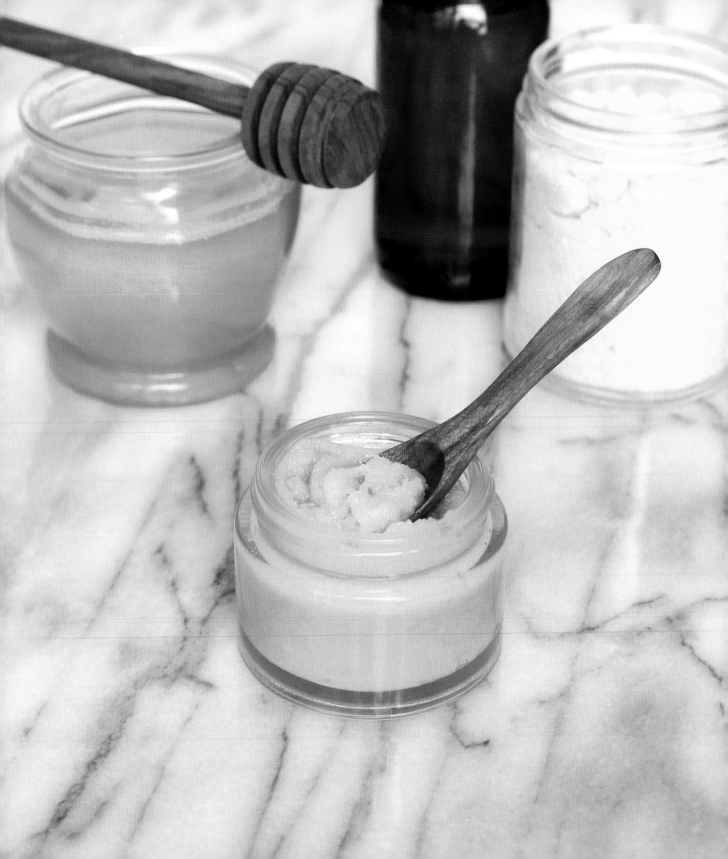

Moisturizing Honey Almond Skin Polish

I just don't know what's sweeter: honey or the way this Moisturizing Honey Almond Skin Polish leaves your face feeling and looking silky smooth.

Almond meal helps to lift dead skin cells up and away while moisturizing the skin with nourishing oils. Honey not only helps fight bacteria but also provides skin with a wash of antioxidants and draws moisture to the skin as a natural humectant. Apricot kernel oil provides more moisture, nourishing the newly exposed layer of skin. The result is ultra-soft skin with an undeniable glow.

YIELD: 4 OZ (120 ML)

4 tbsp (28 g) finely ground almond meal

2 tbsp (30 ml) raw honey

1 tbsp (15 ml) apricot kernel oil

In a small bowl, mix all the ingredients together into a smooth paste.

Store the paste in a small, airtight jar and use as needed.

To use, place a small scoop of the skin polish in the palm of your hand and add a few drops of warm water. Simply stir the water and the polish together in your palm, using your finger, and then rub into the face using gentle, circular motions.

Wash off with warm water and follow with moisturizer.

Siren Seaweed Mask

You may recall from your high school Greek mythology lesson that sirens were beautiful sea creatures that captivated and lured sailors to their deaths. I think it's a safe bet that they had amazing skin! Perhaps they knew the power of seaweed.

Seaweed is the star of this mask: It infuses skin with vitamins and minerals while stimulating the production of collagen. Chlorella is a sea algae that is rich in the antioxidant vitamin A as well as zinc. Yogurt is the perfect base, as some of the skin-loving goodies in seaweed are water-soluble, while others are oil-soluble. Plus, the lactic acid in yogurt is a mild exfoliant, stimulating collagen production and leaving skin super soft and siren-worthy.

YIELD: 1 MASK

2 tsp (10 ml) full-fat, plain yogurt

1 drop rose, geranium or ylang-ylang essential oil

¼ tsp kelp powder

¼ tsp chlorella powder

In a small bowl, mix the drop of essential oil into the yogurt base.

Add the kelp and chlorella, and mix until you have a smooth consistency.

Apply a generous layer of the mask, and let it sit for 10 to 15 minutes. (Do feel free to practice your siren song at this time.)

Rinse off with warm water and apply moisturizer.

NOTES

This mask has a tiny bit of an odd odor but it's a small price to pay, in my opinion! The essential oil does help mask the scent slightly, so if your nose is particularly sensitive, don't skip out on that ingredient!

Since this mask mildly exfoliates the skin, use it no more than once or twice a week to avoid irritation. Any redness should subside within a few minutes to an hour after washing the mask off.

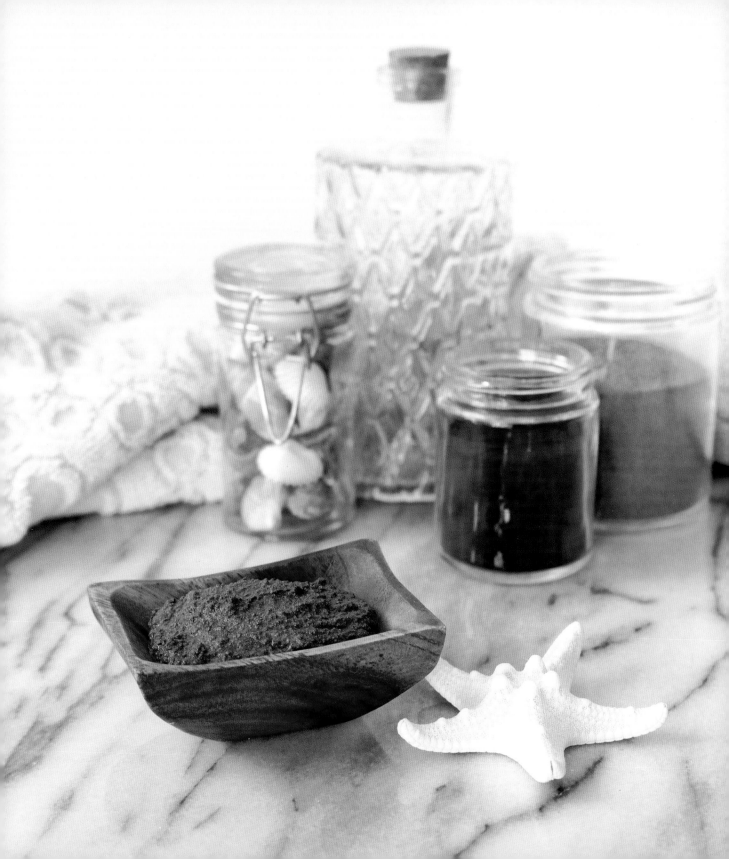

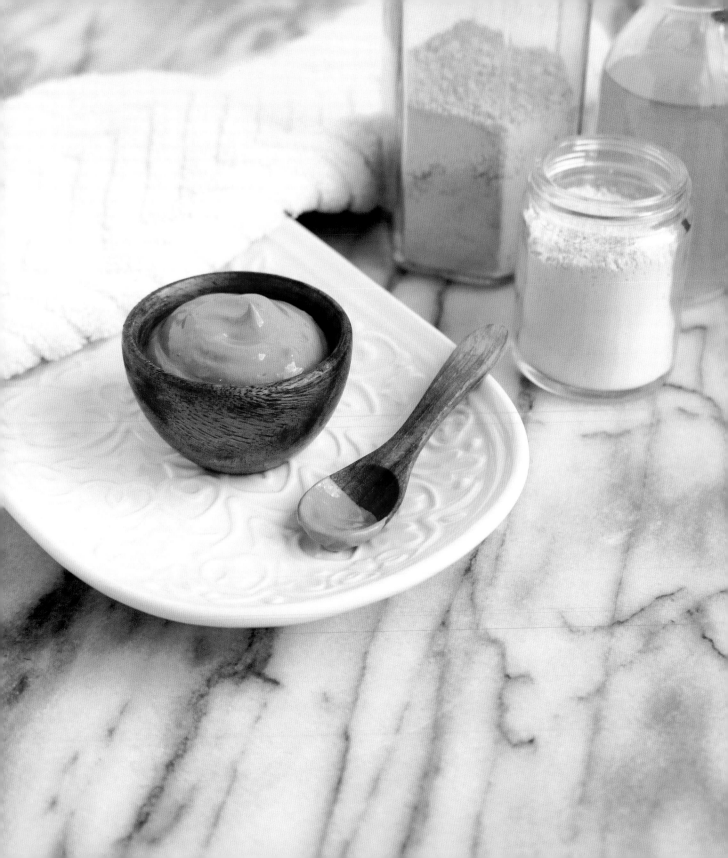

Pore-Perfecting Clay Mask

The green clay mask is iconic—a skincare classic. And for good reason! Clays are not only filled with skin-loving minerals, they also help to draw oil and impurities from pores.

This particular mask is especially great for those suffering from breakouts and excessively oily skin. Bentonite clay and French green clay both provide skin with vital minerals while helping to draw impurities and oil from the pores. Apple cider vinegar balances the skin's pH and helps keep unwanted bacteria in check.

YIELD: 1 MASK

1 tsp (3 g) bentonite clay

1 tsp (3 g) French green clay

1 tsp (5 ml) water

1 tsp (5 ml) apple cider vinegar

In a small bowl, mix all ingredients together into a smooth paste.

Apply a thick layer of the mask to clean, slightly damp skin.

Allow the mask to sit for 5 to 10 minutes, and then wash off with warm water.

NOTE: To prevent skin from getting irritated, remove the mask before it dries completely. Any tightness or itchiness are signs that the mask is drying and ready to be washed off.

Protecting Matcha Mask

Matcha is to green tea as the Hulk is to Bruce Banner: it's the superpowerful, lime green version. And just like the Hulk, matcha provides superhero protection (except without that whole anger management issue).

With ten times the antioxidants as classic green tea, matcha helps neutralize DNA-damaging free radicals and prevent skin sebum from oxidizing. As natural humectants, the raw honey and aloe help to draw moisture to the skin, keeping it hydrated and healthy looking.

YIELD: 1 MASK

1 tsp (5 ml) raw honey

½ tsp aloe vera gel

1 tsp (1 g) matcha green tea powder

In a small bowl, mix all the ingredients together into a smooth paste.

Apply to clean skin and let sit for 10 to 15 minutes.

Wash off and follow with moisturizer.

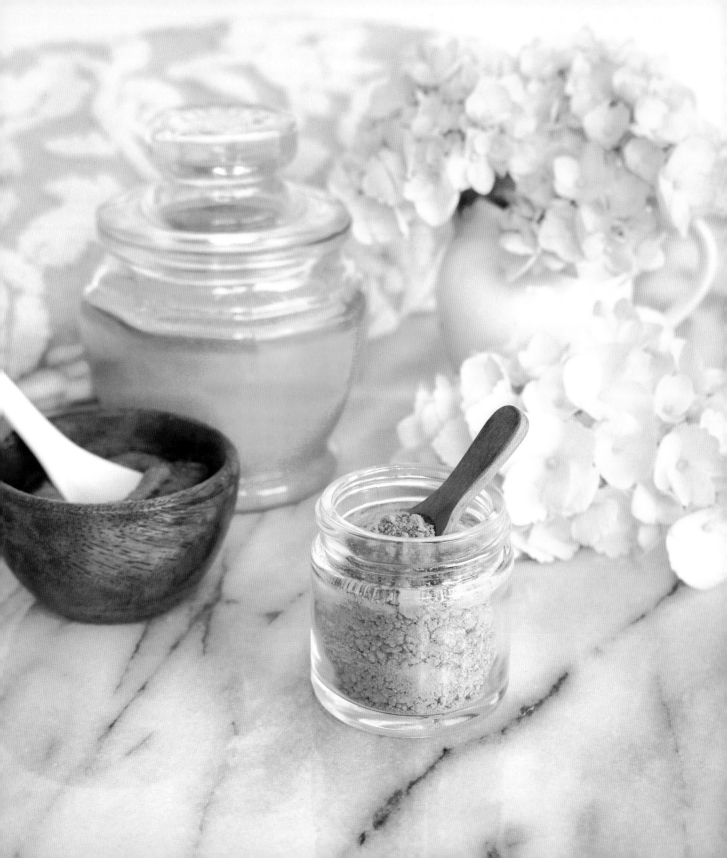

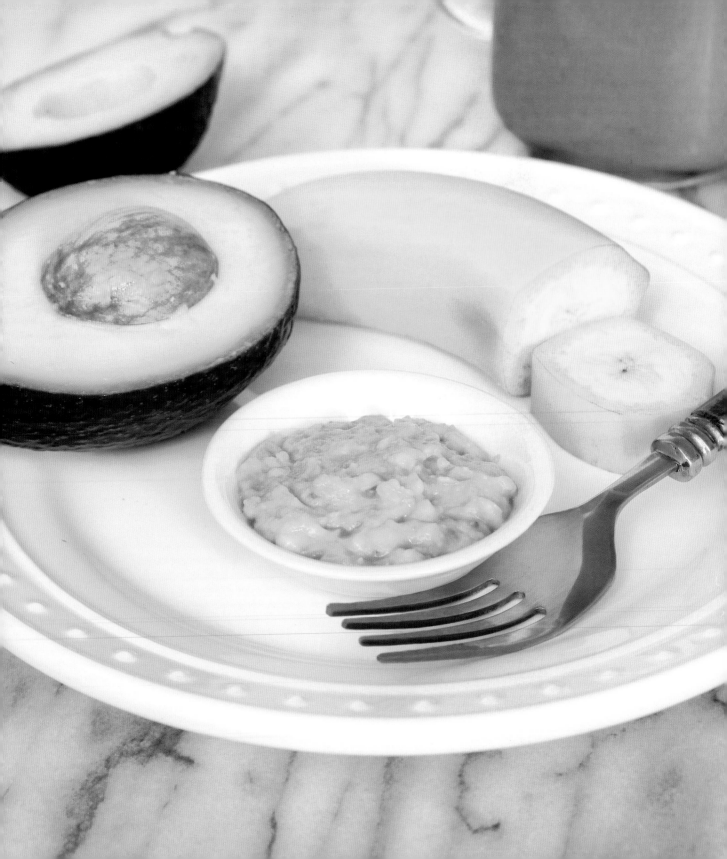

Moisturizing Avo-Nana Mask

The next time you're making yourself a green smoothie, take a second to try this mask while you're at it—simply portion off a little avocado and banana, combine them, rub the mixture on your face and carry on with your smoothie-making business like the multitasking glow-getter you are.

Avocado provides the skin with rich moisture as well as critical vitamins and minerals, especially the antioxidant vitamin E. Banana similarly helps moisturize and is filled with glow-getting nutrients. Together they deliver a smooth, hydrated, glowing complexion.

YIELD: 1 MASK

1 tsp (5 g) mashed avocado

1 tsp (6 g) mashed banana

In a small bowl, combine the avocado and banana and mix into a smooth and consistent paste.

Apply the mask to clean skin and allow it to sit for 10 to 15 minutes.

Wash off and follow with moisturizer.

Favorite Face Oil for All Skin Types

This face oil blend is one-size-fits-most, filled with carrier and essential oils that tend to do well with a range of skin types. The blend moisturizes deeply yet sinks right into the skin, soothes irritations and is filled with critical vitamins.

Grapeseed oil is one of the most widely loved oils by individuals of all skin types. Pumpkin seed oil feeds the skin from the outside with moisturizing essential fatty acids, the antioxidant vitamins A and C, and zinc. Jojoba oil is very similar to the skin's natural sebum, quickly absorbing into the skin and helping to balance the skin's own oil production.

YIELD: 2 OZ (60 ML)

2 tbsp (30 ml) grapeseed oil

1 tbsp (15 ml) pumpkin seed oil

1 tbsp (15 ml) jojoba oil

4 drops lavender essential oil

4 drops geranium essential oil

4 drops frankincense essential oil

In a 2-ounce (60-ml) glass dropper bottle, combine all the ingredients and shake well.

Apply 4 to 6 drops to your entire face.

NOTE: The ingredients will sink into your skin rather quickly, but if applying makeup, you may want to wait a few minutes.

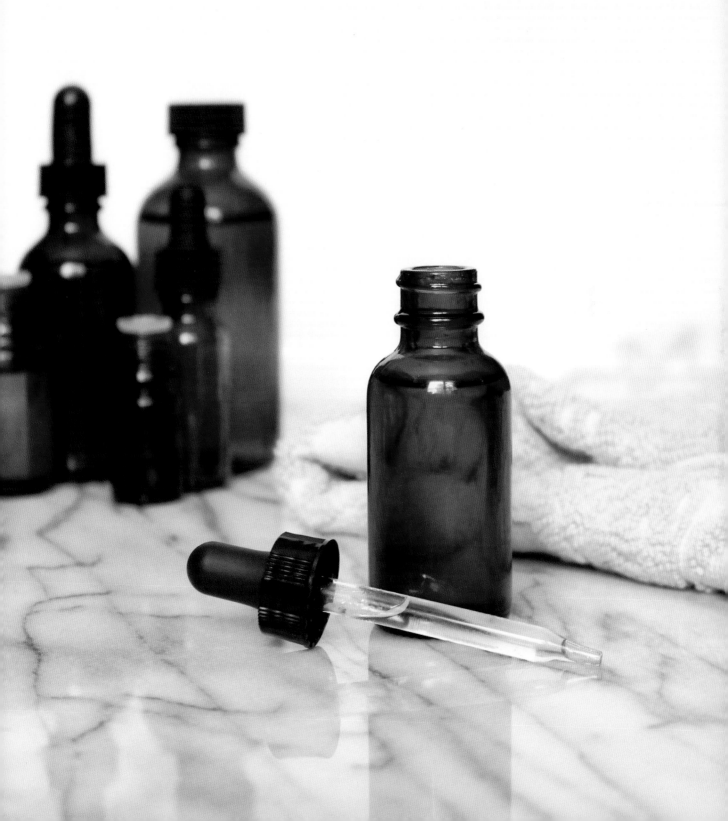

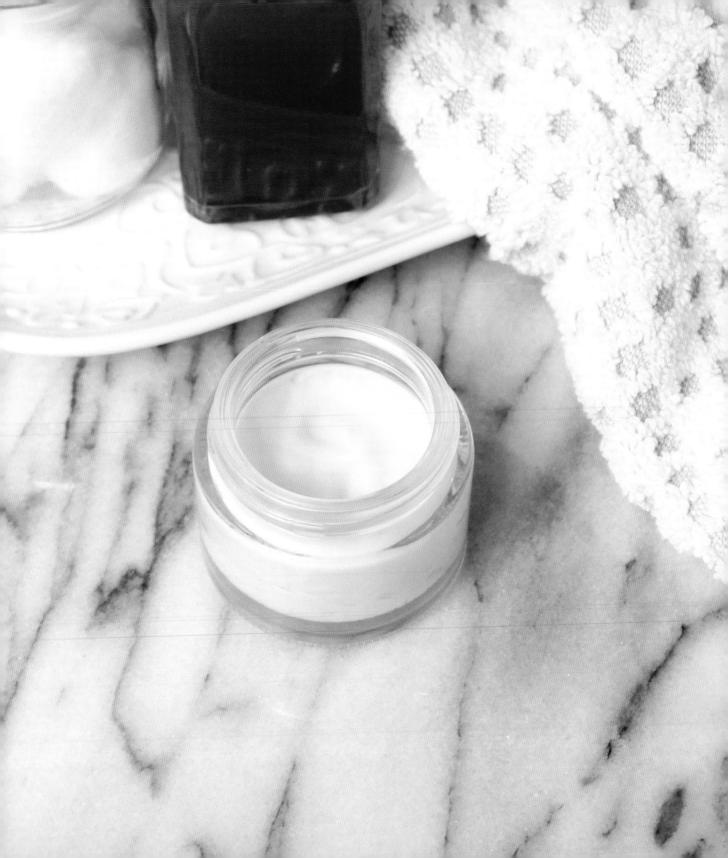

Ultramoisturizing Lotion

If your skin is parched, this lotion is the tall glass of water it's been asking for. It provides the skin with a perfect balance of moisture from both water (thanks to the aloe) and lipids (thanks to the shea butter and grapeseed oil). As a natural humectant, vegetable glycerin draws water close and keeps it locked in the skin where it is needed. The result is an unbelievably soft complexion. Like butter. Like velvet. Like a baby's bottom. Like something you just want to touch all day long. In all seriousness though, prepare to find yourself delicately stroking your own face as you would a puppy's perfect little head.

YIELD: 2 OZ (60 ML)

1 tbsp (14 g) shea butter

2 tsp (10 ml) grapeseed oil

2 tbsp (30 ml) aloe vera gel

⅛ tsp vegetable glycerin

8 drops lavender essential oil

4 drops rosemary essential oil

4 drops frankincense essential oil

In the top of a double boiler, melt the shea butter. Once it is melted, remove it from the heat and let it cool for a few minutes.

After the shea butter has cooled a bit, add the grapeseed oil. Stir to combine. Let the mixture solidify for at least 2 hours.

After the mixture has solidified a bit, add the aloe, glycerin and essential oils. Stir everything together vigorously until the lotion is one even consistency.

Use a small amount whenever desired!

NOTES

Don't have a double boiler? No problem! Simply simmer a few inches (centimeters) of water in a saucepan, and then place a heatproof bowl on top of the saucepan. The steam will heat the bowl and melt your ingredients.

Oil and water don't like to mix, so the ingredients may separate a bit once they've settled. If you happen to have emulsifying wax on hand, adding ¼ teaspoon during the first step will prevent this from happening. But it's not necessary—though the lotion may look atypical, it will do exactly what it is supposed to once applied to your skin!

This lotion isn't just great for the face! Slather it on stubborn dry spots and hands.

Hydrating Rose Facial Mist

This facial mist is as pleasurable as it is effective. It smells downright divine and hydrates the skin with two powerful natural humectants, aloe vera and vegetable glycerin. Just close your eyes and pretend you're standing next to a magical, rose-scented waterfall that transforms your skin into dewy perfection.

If you're a fan of face oils as I am, this mist is a great way to hydrate your skin with the power of humectants before applying your oil. It's also great for a midday hydration boost—especially during drying winter months—and for countering dehydrating airplane air while traveling.

YIELD: 2 OZ (60 ML)

3 tbsp (45 ml) rose water

2 tsp (10 ml) aloe vera gel

1 tsp (5 ml) vegetable glycerin

In a 2-ounce (60-ml) glass spray bottle, combine all ingredients and shake well.

Close your eyes and spray 1 to 3 times 6 to 10 inches (15 to 25.5 cm) from your face.

NOTE: Vegetable glycerin can leave skin feeling a little sticky. If you find that this recipe is too sticky for daytime wear, dilute the mixture with more rose water and be sure to reduce the amount of vegetable glycerin included next time.

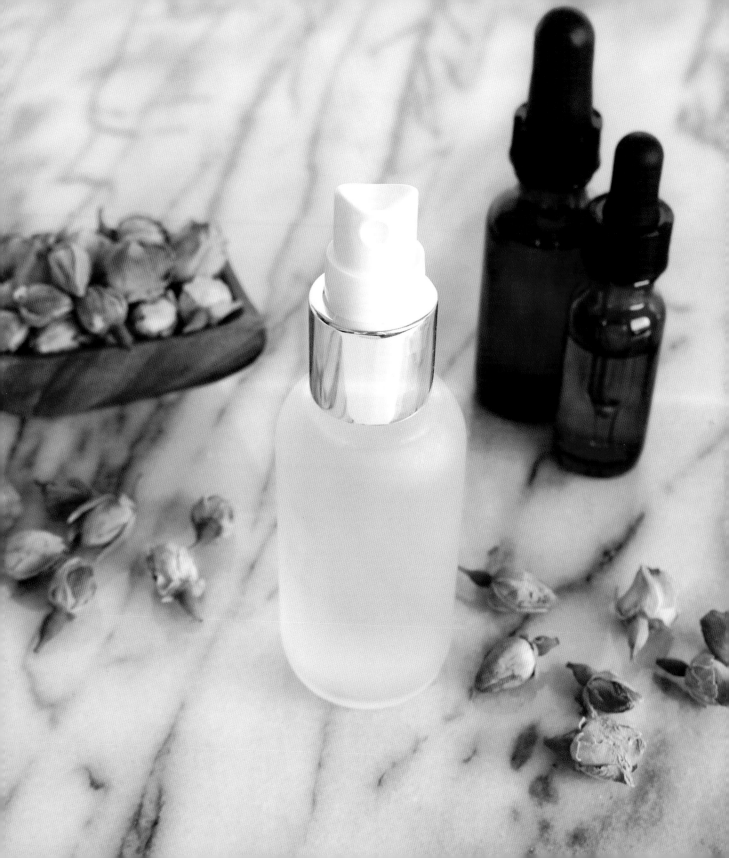

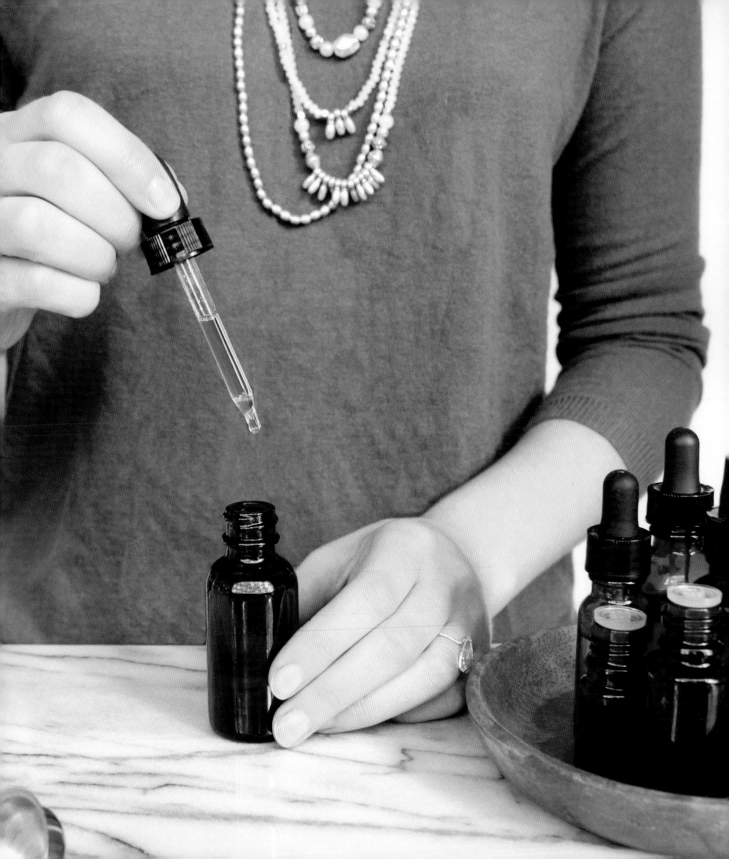

Youth Serum Face Oil for Aging/Mature Skin

Just as our wardrobe, hairdos and opinions evolve over time, so should our skincare. Because the skin's needs change as we age—cell turnover decreases and skin becomes drier, causing skin to look dull and even more aged than it really is. This Youth Serum Face Oil contains ingredients that specifically help address these changes.

Rosehip seed oil is rich in free radical–fighting antioxidants, especially vitamin C. For this reason, it is prized for increasing cell turnover and smoothing skin. Apricot kernel oil is amazingly moisturizing without leaving skin greasy or shiny. It's also rich in antioxidants, boosting the protective power of the serum. Carrot seed, lavender and frankincense essential oils are each fantastic for aging and mature skin, improving cell turnover as well as skin tone and elasticity.

YIELD: 2 OZ (60 ML)

2 tbsp (30 ml) rosehip seed oil

2 tbsp (30 ml) apricot kernel oil

8 drops carrot seed essential oil

6 drops lavender essential oil

6 drops frankincense essential oil

In a 2-ounce (60-ml) glass dropper bottle, combine all the ingredients and shake well.

Apply 4 to 6 drops to your entire face.

Calming Chamomile and Calendula–Infused Oil

This oil is like a much-needed, weeklong beach vacation (complete with daily massages and plenty of mai tais) for skin that is irritated, ornery and stressed out.

Both chamomile and calendula have long been used in traditional medicine for soothing skin irritations and promoting skin healing. Calendula is also antiseptic and anti-inflammatory, boosting its benefits for chapped and irritated skin. Apricot kernel oil provides rich moisture that aids healing while quickly absorbing into the skin. Thanks to this trio of all-star ingredients, this oil can help soothe skin irritated by eczema, razor burn or dermatitis.

YIELD: 3 OZ (90 ML)

½ cup (120 ml) apricot kernel oil

4 tbsp (8 g) dried chamomile flowers

4 tbsp (8 g) dried calendula flowers

In an airtight glass jar, combine all ingredients. Give the ingredients a little shake to allow the oil to saturate the dried flowers.

Place the jar on a well-lit windowsill and allow to steep for 2 weeks.

After 2 weeks of steeping, strain the chamomile and calendula from the oil, using cheesecloth or a coffee filter.

Store the oil in a glass jar or bottle, and use when needed.

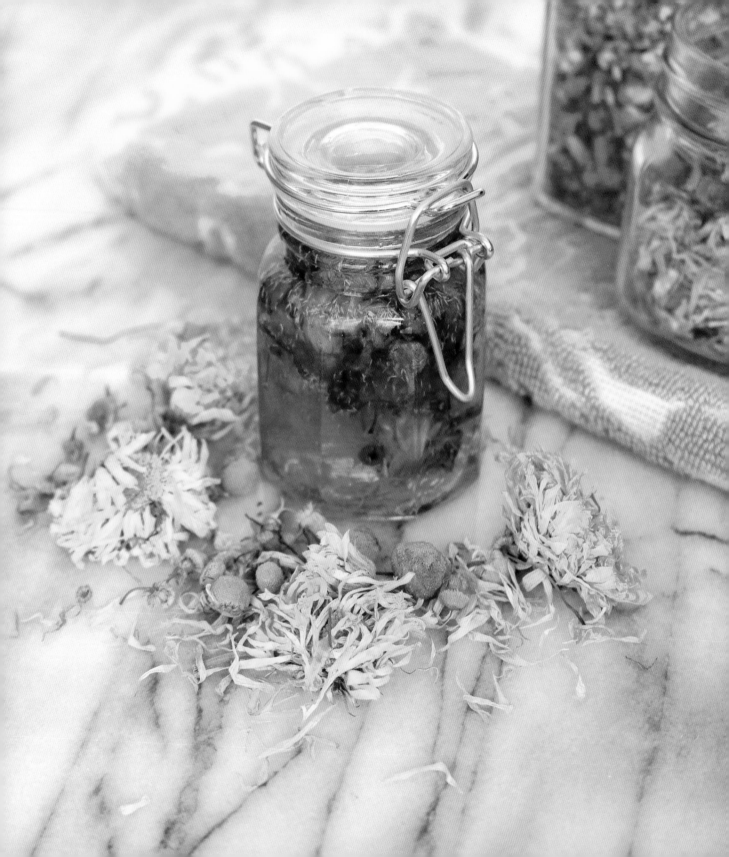

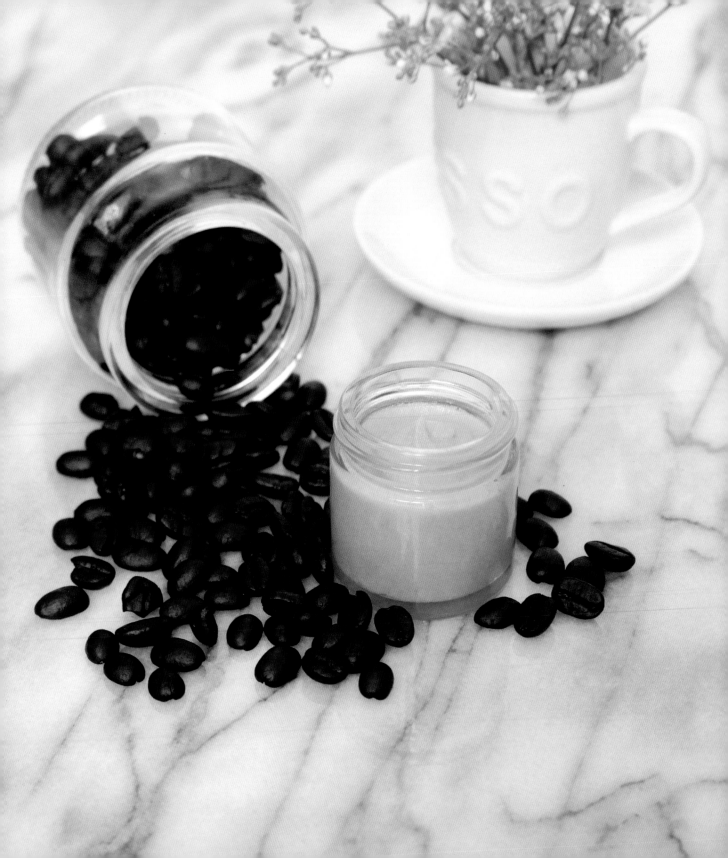

Brightening Coffee-Infused Caffeine Eye Cream

Just as the smell of coffee is sure to perk you up in the morning, the pungent little black bean has the same effect on your skin. This is because caffeine increases the microcirculation of blood in the skin. Coffee also has antioxidant properties, helping protect cells against free radical damage and slow the process of photoaging.

Shea butter and avocado oil are also packed with antioxidants and extremely moisturizing to boot, helping to fight collagen-damaging free radicals and smooth the appearance of fine lines and wrinkles.

YIELD: 1 OZ (30 ML)

1 tbsp (5 g) ground coffee beans

2 tbsp (30 ml) avocado oil

1 tbsp (14 g) shea butter

½ tsp beeswax pastilles

In a heatproof mason jar, combine the ground coffee beans and avocado oil and cover with a lid.

To infuse the oil, heat it low and slow for 5 hours, using either a slow cooker or the stovetop:

For the slow cooker, fill the crock with 2 inches (5 cm) of water, place the jar in the crock and set the cooker on low.

For the stovetop, fill a small pot with 2 inches (5 cm) of water and place the jar in the pot over low heat (the water should be consistently steaming but not boiling). If using this method, be sure to keep an eye on it. You may need to add a little more water at some point.

After 5 hours, turn off the slow cooker or burner and remove the jar. Allow the jar to sit for an hour to cool.

Strain the coffee grounds from the infused oil, using cheesecloth or a coffee filter. Give the grounds a squeeze to get as much oil out as possible, but don't worry about getting every last drop—the recipe accounts for only being able to strain about half.

In the top of a double boiler, melt the beeswax. After the wax has melted, add the shea butter. Once the shea butter has melted, add the infused avocado oil. Stir to combine and pour in a small jar.

Allow the cream to cool and set before using.

NOTE: Avocado and coconut oil are the only two oils I heat to infuse, since they're more molecularly stable than other face oils.

Smoothing Eye Cream

The skin around the eyes is the most thin and delicate on the whole body, which is why it's one of the first areas to show signs of aging. So, it deserves some extra TLC!

This Smoothing Eye Cream is loaded with ingredients that help protect the delicate skin around the eyes and slow the signs of aging. Kokum butter is most often used to treat dry and damaged skin. Shea butter is extremely moisturizing and rich in the antioxidants vitamins A, C and E, which help protect the skin from free radical damage as well as increase cell turnover and collagen production. Rosehip oil and carrot seed essential oil also help to increase cellular turnover.

YIELD: 1 OZ (30 ML)

1 tsp (4 g) kokum butter

1 tsp (5 g) shea butter

1 tsp (5 g) rosehip oil

5 drops carrot seed essential oil

In the top of a double boiler, melt the kokum and shea butters. Once they are melted, remove the mixture from the heat and let it cool for a few minutes.

Add the rosehip oil and carrot seed essential oil to the mixture and stir.

Allow the cream to set for at least 2 hours.

Delicately dab a small amount of the cream around your eye area.

NOTE: Don't have a double boiler? No problem! Simply simmer a few inches (centimeters) of water in a saucepan, and then place a heatproof bowl on top of the saucepan. The steam will heat the bowl and melt your ingredients.

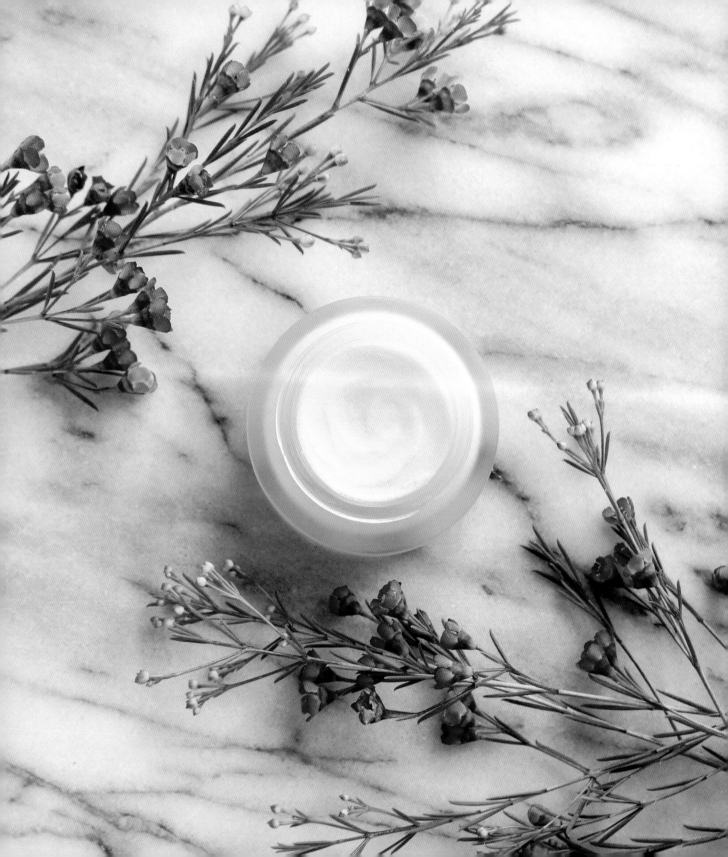

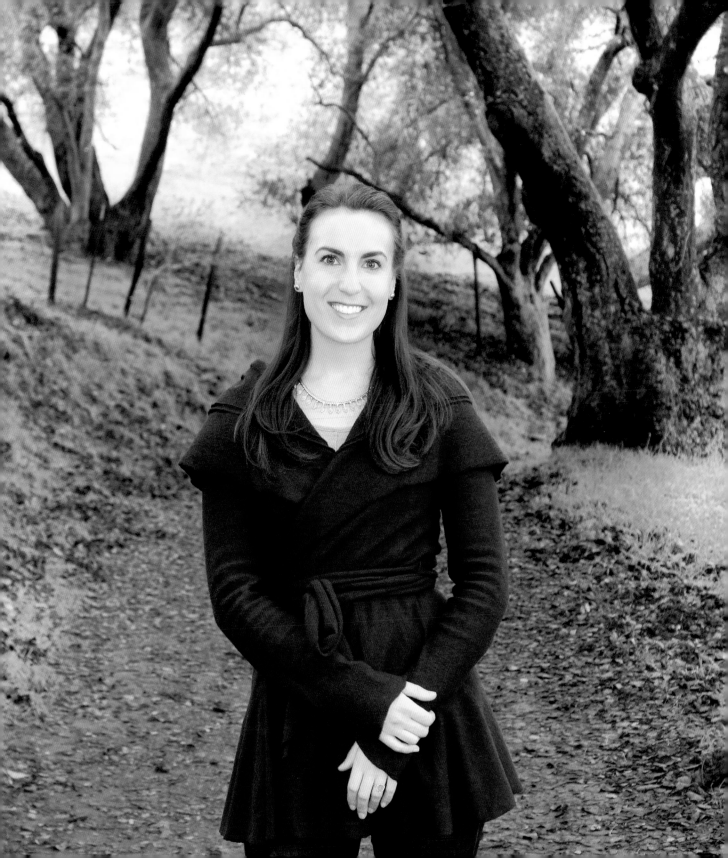

Acknowledgments

• • •

To Body Unburdened's dedicated readers: You have played such an important role in my own health journey and I am humbled to have played a part in yours. Your endless curiosity and passion for natural skincare inspired me to write this book.

To my editor Sarah Monroe and the rest of the Page Street team: You have been so patient with all of my last-minute edits, first-time-author anxiety and control freakery. I am extremely grateful for this wonderful opportunity and to have worked with such a smart, encouraging team.

To my sister Natasha Groff, my sister-in-law Emily Neumann, and my sister-from-another-mister Emily Greenberg: You are the most amazing friends. Thank you for your unending support and always lending your honest opinions.

To my parents: You have provided a lifetime of encouragement and support. Words alone cannot express my gratitude.

To my husband, Eric: You are everything to me. And I don't just mean as my assistant photographer, recipe tester, DIY guinea pig, sounding board, comic relief, number one cheerleader and pillar of strength. You make everything worth celebrating feel one hundred times more wonderful. (P.S. I'm sorry for all the times you had to deal with an entire kitchen full of food that was off limits because it had yet to be photographed.)

About the Author

• • •

Nadia Neumann is the founder of the popular health and wellness website Body Unburdened, where she empowers readers to live a healthy lifestyle rooted in real food, natural beauty and a nontoxic home. She holds a BA in international relations from Boston College and is a Nutritional Therapy Practitioner (NTP™) certified by the Nutritional Therapy Association.

When she's not busy writing or perfecting her face oil blends, Nadia enjoys hiking, spending hours in front of a puzzle, finding new ways to sneak more cacao into her diet and fantasizing about her future garden. A New Jersey native, Nadia currently lives in San Jose, California, with her husband, Eric.

Index

• • •

Chamomile

Calming Chamomile Aloe Face Toner, 153

Calming Chamomile and Calendula Infused Oil, 178

Chamomile Rose Cleansing Grains, 146

Chemical exposure, 10, 73, 123–127

Chemical industry, 125

Chewing, 50

Chia seeds, 60

Berry Satisfying Chia Pudding Parfait, 99

Chicken: Curried Avocado Chicken Salad, 84

Chicken skin, 21

Chili, Sweet and Savory Butternut Squash Chili, 88

Chronic inflammation, 10, 30, 33, 58, 60, 61

Clays, 131, 146, 165

Cleansers

Chamomile Rose Cleansing Grains, 146

Like-Dissolves-Like Cleansing OIl, 149

Nourishing Honey Face Wash, 145

Cleansing, 137–139

Cobalamin, 39

Coca's pulse test, 66–67

Coconut, 57

Coconutty Energy Bites, 107

Tropical Turmeric Ice Pops, 112

Coconut milk

Beet and Berry Smoothie, 115

Berry Satisfying Chia Pudding Parfait, 99

Nadia's Go-to Green Smoothie, 100

Simple Homemade Coconut Milk, 120

Coconut oil, 34

Coconut sugar, 48

Coffee, 35

Collagen, 18, 20, 28, 45, 63

Complete proteins, 27

Concealer, 9

Copper, 40

Corn oil, 60

Corn syrup, 46

Cortisol, 66, 71–73, 79

Cucumbers, 91

Curcumin, 63

D

Dairy products

acne and, 72

avoidance of, 34

grain-fed, 34

raw grass-fed, 27, 34

Dandelion root, 76

Dermatitis, 49, 58

Dermis, 18, 20

Detoxification, 54, 73–76, 79

Detox reactions, 13, 68

Diet

balanced, 79

elimination, 67–70

healthy skin and, 10–12

processed foods in modern, 23, 24

real food, 24–25

Diethanolamine (DEA), 126

Digestive system, 45, 49–57, 78

"Dirty hormones," 73, 75

Diuretics, 35

Dopamine, 47

Dressings

Blueberry Balsamic Dressing, 95

Sweet and Spicy Dressing, 91

Drinking, while eating, 52

Dry skin, 21

E

Eating, drinking while, 52

Eczema, 21, 42, 49, 58

Eggs

from pasture-raised hens, 27

Sweet Pepper Mini Frittatas, 96

Elastin, 18, 20, 45

Electrolytes, 35

Elimination diet, 67–70

Endocrine disrupters, 10, 73, 134

Endocrine system, 75, 76

Environmental pollution, 127, 133, 135

Environmental Working Group, 128

Epidermis, 18

Essential fatty acids (EFAs), 27, 31, 60–61, 83

Essential oils, 131, 145, 149, 157, 170, 173, 177

Estrogens, 71

Exfoliation, 135, 139

Moisturizing Honey Almond Skin Polish, 161

Shockingly Simple At-Home Microdermabrasion, 158

Eye creams

Brightening Coffee-Infused Caffeine Eye Cream, 181

Smoothing Eye Cream, 182

F

Face masks, 139

Moisturizing Avo-Nana Mask, 169

Pore-Perfecting Clay Mask, 165

Protecting Matcha Mask, 166

Siren Seaweed Mask, 162

Face wash. *See* Cleansers

Face washing, 137–139

Factory farms, 27

Fats, 31–35, 47, 75, 78

Fat-soluble vitamins, 31, 36, 40–41, 53

Fermented vegetables, 57

Fiber, 28, 54, 75

Fish

Herbed Sardine Cakes, 87